To Karen,

　　Happy 15th Birthday
from your "Weight Watching"
Aunt Ruthie!

　　　　　August 6, 1983

The Woman Doctor's Diet for Teen-Age Girls

Barbara Edelstein, M.D.

The Woman Doctor's Diet for Teen-Age Girls

PRENTICE-HALL, INC., Englewood Cliffs, N.J.

The Woman Doctor's Diet for Teen-Age Girls
by Barbara Edelstein, M.D.
Copyright © 1980 by Barbara Edelstein, M.D., P.C.
All rights reserved. No part of this book may be
reproduced in any form or by any means, except
for the inclusion of brief quotations in a review,
without permission in writing from the publisher.
Printed in the United States of America
Prentice-Hall International, Inc., London
Prentice-Hall of Australia, Pty. Ltd., Sydney
Prentice-Hall of Canada, Ltd., Toronto
Prentice-Hall of India Private Ltd., New Delhi
Prentice-Hall of Japan, Inc., Tokyo
Prentice-Hall of Southeast Asia Pte. Ltd., Singapore
Whitehall Books Limited, Wellington, New Zealand
10 9 8 7 6 5 4 3 2 1

Library of Congress Cataloging in Publication Data
Edelstein, Barbara.
The woman doctor's diet for teen-age girls.
Includes index.
SUMMARY: Defines overweight, discusses its importance and causes, suggests diets, and gives advice on
dieting with the special physical and social needs of
teenage girls in mind.
1. Obesity in children—Juvenile literature.
2. Reducing diets—Juvenile literature. 3. Adolescent girls—Nutrition—Juvenile literature.
[1. Weight control. 2. Obesity] I. Title.
RJ399.C6E38 1980   613.2'5   79-26546
ISBN 0-13-961631-4

To my wonderful dad, Dr. Howard Fiedler—a great psychiatrist—who came out of retirement and "practice sat" while I wrote this book. He ended up stealing the hearts of all my patients, but I couldn't lose to a nicer guy.

To my charming mother, Roselyn Fiedler, who agreed to leave sunny Florida to "kid sit" so that the grandchildren would at least "get a decent meal."

With love

Acknowledgments

To my son, David, age 20, who did the impossible by editing his mother's book and carried it off with impeccable style and expertise.

To: Lois Shea—Conard High School
    Ann Reinsmith—Sedgwick School
    Parker Simmonds—Bugbee School
    Bernice Maxwell—Avon School
    Pauline Frey—Tolland School
    Nancy Jurkowski—Enrico Fermi High School
    Sister Evelyn O'Connor—St. Augustine's School
    Gay Amato—Duffy School
    Janice Clark—Vernon "Trim Teens"
    Elisa Alter—Hall High School
    Davidsons—Clancy's

Progressive people in progressive schools who shared ideas and feelings with me and allowed me to get "in touch" with the many female teen-agers.

To Heidi Edelstein, age 13, who gave up comic books and TV to be my first reader and teen consultant.

To Jackie Landry, my marvelous nurse, who held the office together with her chewing gum and personality while I was in hibernation.

Contents

Introduction

Close to 90 percent of my fat adult patients were once fat teen-agers. After fifteen years of watching their struggle to lose weight, and after writing a book—*The Woman Doctor's Diet for Women*—to help them do it, I decided that my next project should be a book for teen-age girls. After a certain age—around 25—it becomes very difficult to *control* overweight; the reason I wrote this book was to help you *prevent* it.

I wanted to offer advice and encouragement to girls who have enough problems without being overweight. I was a fat teen-ager myself, and I know how difficult it is to handle everything that gets thrown at you from ages 12 to 20. True, I grew up at a time when there wasn't the emphasis on being thin that there is today—but it was bad enough.

There were no tent dresses, no elastic waistbands, and no diet salad dressings. How I hated those princess-style dresses and salads with vinegar or lemon juice. How I hated hearing people (especially my mother) say, "You would be so pretty if you would only lose 10 pounds." (I was 5 feet 3 inches and weighed about 130 pounds.)

Like many of you, I tried various methods to lose weight, usually crash diets. None of them made much sense, and I always ended up with hollow cheeks and circles under my eyes, but the same chubby knees and heavy legs (that's the crash diet look). My first diet consisted solely of eggs and skim milk, blended together. It was horrible. The second diet let me eat 12 oranges a day and a soup made of cabbage, tomatoes, and carrots without salt. That one left me weak and tired. Then I tried a milky, liquid "balanced diet" from a can. It gave me terrible gas pains, and I was doubled over for two weeks. I assumed that dieting meant being in agony.

Looking back, I wish there had been someone to answer my questions:

1. Why me? What did I do to deserve my weight? I don't eat that much.
2. Are all diets the same? What's the best diet for me at my present age (between 12 and 20)? Will I need a different diet 5 years from now?
3. What should I know about nutrition and exercise to help me make decisions about how I should lose weight?
4. How can I diet without killing myself?
5. What's going to happen to me while I'm dieting? To my body? To my mind?
6. What will life be like if I do get thin? How will people react to me? Do I have to diet for the rest of my life?

I wish someone had answered these and other questions and had cleared up all my misconceptions.

That was a long time ago, and many teen-agers still have the same questions, fears, and misconceptions. The difference is that now, instead of no available dieting information, there is an incredible volume of *mis*information. And it's no longer just *nice* to be thin; it's considered a *must*, a way of life.

Mothers are constantly torn between wanting their daughters to be super thin and worrying about their being well-fed and well-nourished. At the first extreme, parents may push their daughters too hard to lose weight, often devising diets that don't take into account the proper nutritional requirements of a growing teen-ager. At the latter extreme, parents may face a painful dilemma: how can they think of denying you food? How can they encourage you to stop eating when they have worked so hard to give you as much as you want? Of course they want to be proud of the way you look, but they may panic if they feel a diet is endangering your health or if they sense that you are suffering too much. They mean well, but they are often confused and misinformed.

"Eat a lot but stay thin," they seem to say. If you have a tendency to be overweight, this can't be done.

The pressure is all around us. There isn't a teen or popular magazine that doesn't run new diets in every issue, or a newspaper that doesn't carry features on weight-control. I've practiced bariatric medicine for 15 years and have talked to hundreds of teen-age girls. There aren't many—fat *or* thin—who aren't concerned about their weight.

But with the glut of crazy crash diets and diet propaganda in our society, it is vital that you, the teen-age girl, learn to make intelligent, informed choices about how to lose weight, when to stop, and how to handle the problems that will inevitably arise at home, in school, among friends, and most important, within your own body. You have to understand why you are overweight and how you can prevent this tendency from interfering with your happiness and success in years to come.

You are teen-age and female, and you need a diet book of your own. You must remember the following things:

1. You can't diet the way your mother does because your body is still changing and your needs are different.
2. You can't diet the way boys do because they have a much easier time losing weight. That's right, boys have it *easy.*

Boys can grow out of baby fat. Girls do not. Remember that fat, blobby Bobby at the desk next to you? At 10 years old he was twice as fat as you. Now at 14 he is suddenly tall and slim. He grew to be 5 feet 7 inches, and somehow you got hung up at 5 feet 4 inches. Perhaps you've told yourself, "I'm not too fat, I'm just too short." Forget it. Chances are you won't grow much taller. And not only will you not "grow out" of your baby fat, you'll probably find it settling in some pretty unsightly places. Maybe if you had realized this at 11 or 12, you wouldn't have gobbled down so many chocolate chip cookies every day or rewarded yourself with a hot fudge sundae or a milk shake after a hard day at school.

Boys can eat twice as much food as girls, burn off twice as much energy doing the same things, and lose weight twice as quickly. You will watch your father and your brothers wolfing down huge quantities of food and not gaining an ounce. And you will see them just as easily drop 10 pounds merely by giving up dessert.

Boys can get away with being fat. Girls cannot. Girls have a much more difficult time socially being overweight. Ever notice some of those football players? They have massive legs, bulky middles, and titanic rear ends. I'd like to see a girl so popular with a rear end like that.

Nature isn't always fair. It's exciting to be a female in an age of greater freedom and equal opportunities, but in terms of weight loss we will always have a much tougher time than men. Girls naturally have twice as much body fat, and instead of burning excess calories the way the male hormones do, your female hormones are dedicated to storing them. Social roles still demand that women purchase and prepare food to feed the family. When a little boy gets a truck for a gift, his sister gets a toy oven. Her association with food is long and insidious.

If you are significantly overweight, your teen years could be the most critical of your life; you will either change your eating habits and struggle to build new priorities and new self-image in a world of irresistible, fattening foods, or else move on as you are to adulthood and a different, more difficult set of dieting problems.

The time to lose weight is *now* while you are younger, more adaptable, more impressionable, and more active.

This book contains many diets that you will find extremely useful. It will help you to lose weight now and to develop the kind of eating habits that will keep you healthy and physically fit for the rest of your life. It is written for *you*, but there are also sections for your parents, family, and friends, people who sometimes get in the way of your diet, but must now be taught to help it succeed. The more people on your side, the greater your chance of success.

And success now will mean far more than it will later. It will give you the strength and self-confidence to overcome the problems that Nature reserves exclusively for its gentler sex, the tougher-than-the-male young woman.

1

Getting Older

Growing Up: Body

I had a tough time growing up 30 years ago, and from what I see and hear, it hasn't gotten any easier. From the first can of deodorant to the first bra to the first tampon, growing up struck me as one embarrassing adjustment after another. But the anticipation is usually more terrifying than what actually happens, like the first ride on a roller coaster: when you reach the highest point you cry, "What am I doing here?"; and when it's all over you wonder, "Why was I so scared?"

You don't grow up overnight. You begin as early as 9 years old, when your breasts begin to show, and end as late as 17, when your periods become regular. It starts when a hormone secreted by the pituitary gland in the brain produces a sudden skeletal or bone growth. Legs and feet reach maximum growth first, which is why adolescent girls often complain that their feet are too big. (The same is true of noses.)

Female growth is usually completed by age 14, at least 2 years earlier than male growth. That's why at junior high school dances most of the girls wear ballet slippers and can rest their chins on their dates' heads. Tall girls shouldn't worry, though: the boys will not only catch up to them, they will generally grow much taller.

A Girl and Her Estrogen

When a girl's period begins, the greatest portion of her skeletal growth is over. At most, she could grow another 2 inches. Once growth has ended and the sexual organs (ovaries) have matured, the process of "feminization" begins. The ovaries begin to manufacture large amounts of estrogen and send it into the bloodstream. It is this estrogen stimulation that causes the breasts to develop and soft curves to appear in the hips, thighs, and rear end. These curves are not an overgrowth of bone, but sex-linked deposits of fat. You're not getting fat (unless you already are), you're just getting female.

Many girls get scared and resist these changes, acting childish or elaborately embarrassed, hiding their bodies under big shirts and loose tent dresses. Others want to speed things up, calling attention to their new femininity with makeup, tight jeans, and low-cut blouses. Timing is also important: nobody wants to be the first to wear a bra, but nobody wants to be the last either.

Initially, the amount of fat deposited in these places depends on the body build that you have inherited from one of your ancestors. You have no control over the size of your breasts or hips; we say that these are *genetically coded*. Even if you get fat during this process, it may not affect your breast size. (It will, however, modify the size of your hips and rear.)

If you refer to the age-height-weight chart in the next chapter, you'll see that even though the period of largest growth is between 11 and 13 in the female, *the period of largest weight gain is between 13 and 18*. At this stage a 2-inch growth can cause a whopping 20-pound gain (at least twice the rate of gain in the growing phase). This is because your estrogens have begun to function, and you are developing an extra layer of fat. Remember, you will have *twice as much body fat as boys*, whether you are overweight or not.

The extra layer of fat is for the purpose of supplying food and protection to your future babies, whether or not you decide to have any. Historically, food supplies have not always been constant—this is Nature's way of insuring the survival of human and animal species at all times.

From this moment on, your estrogen becomes one of the most important physical influences in your life, particularly affecting:

1. *Breasts.* Estrogen plays an important role in breast development, which can start as early as age 9 but is often not completed until 5 or

6 years later. Normally, the breasts go through five stages—infantile, budding, first enlargement, formation of a mound around the nipple, and final enlargement—before they reach adult size, and each stage is dependent on estrogen.

2. *Pelvis.* Even though you are born with a wider pelvis than boys (for having children), it is estrogen that causes it to assume adult proportions. Not only does the pelvic bone itself enlarge, but estrogen stimulates the deposit of fat around the hips and the tops of legs.

3. *Periods.* The regularity, intensity, and duration of your periods are mainly a function of estrogen. When levels of this hormone are altered because of a change in body size or fat composition, periods become irregular and may even stop for a short time.

4. *Fat.* Estrogen is important in maintaining body fat. Since the female's biological role is to have children, Nature protects that extra layer by promoting the conversion of food into fat.

5. *Fluid Retention and Mood.* Estrogen plays an important role in fluid retention, which causes a bloated feeling and swelling of the breasts the week before a period. This can also affect your mood. Certain English schools determined that poor behavior, lateness, irritability and inattention were greatest the week before menstruation. Appetite may also be increased.

6. *"Youthfulness."* Estrogen keeps your skin elastic, your bones hard, and your body tissue strong. You might say that it keeps you physically young. Your body stops manufacturing estrogen in your late fifties. Doctors once thought that by taking large amounts of estrogen, older women could slow the aging process. While it can keep skin from drying out and bones from crumbling, estrogen also may increase one's chances of getting cancer of the uterus.

Meanwhile, what's happening to boys while you are growing fatter? They are getting *leaner*. Their hormone, testosterone, promotes muscle-building and fat-burning. It also increases the width of their shoulders, deepens their voices, and promotes hair growth on their faces and bodies.

Growing Up: Mind

When I was in psychiatric training, we had a very successful diagnosis for teen-agers called "Adjustment Reaction of Adolescence." This is the transition from the world of childhood to the world of adulthood and is marked by confusing and often frightening physical, hormonal, and intellectual changes. At no other time in your life is it normal...

to laugh one minute and cry the next
to love and hate yourself at the same time

to sneak a cigarette and scream at your mother for smoking
to closet yourself in a room yet long for companionship
to blast your stereo at nerve-shattering levels
to stay on the phone for hours
to contemplate, life, death, suicide, occultism, and political aggression
as logical behavior
to think one minute everyone is looking at you, and the next minute
worry everyone is ignoring you

A weight problem is one more tremendous emotional burden at a time when you have enough to worry about.

Most fears about growing up don't come from physical changes in your body but from the uncertainty about what those changes may bring. Erik Erickson defined the major task of adolescence as the formation of an identity, which depends heavily on peer acceptance and appropriate adult models to copy. This identity allows the adolescent to see herself as independent of her parents, capable of harboring thoughts and ideas different from theirs. She becomes particularly conscious of her past, her social background, and her future place in society.

The most important questions become: Who am I? How will people act toward me? Will my parents keep taking care of me? Will boys like me? Will other girls like me? Relationships that have always been taken for granted have to be questioned and reexamined. The world that was once an extended family (which included parents, grandparents, aunts and uncles, brothers, sisters, and friends) becomes less secure. You realize that life goes through phases, that nothing stays the same.

This is the time when you form a satisfactory or unsatisfactory body image. You look carefully at your appearance, comparing yourself to others. Many times the comparison is unfavorable. You don't like what you see—perhaps you realize that you are fat.

I used to get angry at skinny women who dieted constantly and complained of how fat they were in their teens. I didn't believe them, and furthermore I didn't see why what they looked like in their teens mattered now. But I have since seen photographs of some of them at ages 12, 15, and 17; and they *were* a little overweight, and this "fatty" image haunts them still.

The body image that you form in your teens can affect your whole personality—the way you feel about yourself and relate to other people.

I have heard about a former Miss America—a stunningly beautiful girl—who went to a psychiatrist because she saw herself as homely and awkward. That was her self-image as an adolescent, and it took many hours of therapy to convince her that she had changed, even after she had won a major beauty contest.

Into this normal turmoil comes a girl with the added burden of being overweight. She usually matures earlier than her friends and feels very alone. She already realizes that she is not the ideal, all-American beauty. Because of her early breast development, she is often the butt of sly comments which she is not emotionally ready to handle. So she wraps her immaturity around her like a cloak, preferring the comfort of the family to the competitive "arena" of males and females. Whether she remains fat or thin, this body image never goes away.

You should use these years to get your body into a shape with which you're satisfied. This doesn't mean being unrealistic about how thin you should be, the shape of your legs, or the size of your breasts. It means that given the diversity of body sizes considered "normal," you fit into that group. You don't have to be at the thinnest, shapeliest end of the list, but you shouldn't be at the other extreme either. Overweight should not be your way of life.

2

What Is Overweight?

Overweight Is Weighing Too Much

Fifteen percent of all teen-agers in this country—between 5 and 6 million—are overweight. I would bet that about 80 percent of them are female.

You can't tell if you're overweight just by getting on a scale—it depends on your age, height, build, how much muscle you have, and where your fat is distributed (all in one spot, or like a smooth blanket over your entire body). If you're a teen-ager, it's especially hard to tell because your body is growing and changing at an extremely fast rate. The stubby 11-year-old girl with the short waist and heavy legs may bloom into the curvy 16-year-old with the slender waist and long, shapely legs.

I once asked a pediatrician friend how he determined if a teen-age girl was overweight (apart from the obvious, 200-pound cases). "I don't do any fancy measurements," he said. "I just lift them up, toss them over my shoulder, and if I get a pain in the groin, they're overweight."

He later admitted using a standard pediatrician's chart and adding or subtracting 5 pounds, depending on body build. I like the first way better—at least it *sounds* imprecise, and the other method can often be misleading: a chart can't look you up and down and sling you over its shoulder.

Somewhere along the way—between ages 9 and 15—you pick up an extra layer of fat that you'll carry for the next 40 years. During that transformation, it is difficult to determine your body "type" because the amount and size of your muscles aren't clear. A potentially fat child may be mistaken for an athletic and muscled one, while a tall and slender child can suddenly develop a round, flabby body.

You are technically "overweight" when you are 10 to 15 percent heavier than "normal," but "normal," as I have implied, is a flexible term for teen-agers. This is the accepted "normal" age-height-weight table for ages 10 through 18.

Your Age	Your Height *(inches)*	Your "Normal" Weight *(pounds)*
10	55	70
11	57	79
12	60	88
13	62	99
14	63	108
15	63	114
16	64	117
17	64	119
18	64	120

If you are taller than the chart's average height for your age, add 5 to 5½ pounds per inch.

If you are older than 18, begin with a base of 100 pounds = 5 feet, and for every inch above that height add 4 to 5 pounds. (For example, if you are 20 years old and 5 feet 3 inches tall, then you should weigh between 112 and 115 pounds.)

You can also add or subtract 10 pounds for certain builds. (For example, if you are 5 feet 3 inches tall and built very small, then your normal weight could be just over 100 pounds. If you have a large build, then you could weigh as much as 125 pounds.)

You can determine your build by measuring two things. The first is your wrists. If you can't close the fingers of one hand all the way around the wrist of the other, chances are you have a larger-than-normal build. The other is your shoulder width. If your shoulders are narrower than 32 inches, you have a small build, and if they are wider than 36 inches you have a large build.

Don't compare your "normal" weight to fashion models' weights. You may read of a sex symbol who's 5 feet 9 inches tall and weighs 115 pounds, dripping wet, and despair because you weigh the same and are 5 or 6 inches shorter. Don't worry. Fashion models starve themselves down to extremely low levels to achieve that lean, hungry look that many clothing designers and photographers find so appealing. Place them beside "normal" people, or look at them in person (the television camera, it is said, adds 10 to 15 pounds), and you'll probably find them rather scrawny.

The chart is imperfect, but it can give you a rough idea of where you stand.

There are other tests of overweight that are not nearly as scientific. One, the most obvious, is looking in the mirror. Just look at yourself in the mirror at all angles, naked and clothed. The mirror is reliable, but how you see yourself sometimes isn't. In the end, you may need a second opinion.

A camera can sometimes give you one. Have someone in your family photograph you in a bathing suit, straight on, from the back, and in profile. No fancy angles or poses—just straight. No fair to suck your tummy in either. Relax and stand naturally—these are for *you*, not your school newspaper. Studying these photographs can be a grim, sobering experience, but it's the one way you can get an objective look at yourself.

Dress size is one of the least accurate ways to tell if you're overweight because many, many chubby girls can get into a size 9 or 11 dress. The junior sizes seem to accommodate a fair amount of excess weight, particularly below the waist. Also, the size 9 of one designer may be very different from another's. Often a dress size will reflect your build rather than your weight.

Overweight Is Having Too Many Fat Cells

Being overweight means having an excess amount of fat in your body compared to the amount of muscle and bone.

Fat is a very specialized type of body tissue and represents stored energy. Nature never wastes food, so anything your body doesn't use up immediately gets stored as fat. One pound of fat represents 3500 calories of stored energy—enough fuel to keep your body running for two to three days. You accumulate too much body fat by eating more food or calories than you burn.

Fat is created in two ways. One way is by enlarging the existing fat cells in the body. It's just like blowing up balloons—each cell becomes progressively more overstuffed. If you get fat this way, you can probably become only 15 to 20 pounds overweight in your lifetime because that is about as much as you can overstuff fat cells.

The other way of getting fat is by increasing the *number* of fat cells in your body. This is far more serious: not only are you capable of getting much fatter, but these new cells never go away.

The *way* in which you get fat has nothing to do with the amount of food you eat. It's in the genes you inherit from your parents—something you're born with. The unlucky people are the ones whose bodies have the ability to create lots of new fat cells, and to create them with ease.

Do you have to become fat just because you inherited the trait? Fortunately, no—but you will have to be extremely careful about what you eat, particularly during certain periods of your life when other body changes make it easier for you to create new fat cells.

The first of these times is when you are a baby. Too late—you didn't exactly have any control over that. If your parents fed you too much of the wrong foods, that is probably one of the reasons you're overweight now. It's not their fault, though. Doctors have told us that fat babies grow into exceptionally intelligent, healthy people. Certainly nourishment plays an important part in the physical and psychological well-being of a baby, but there is a difference between a nutritional, well-balanced diet and one with an excessive amount of calories, particularly in the form of carbohydrates and sugar.

Many nutritionists become enraged over this point, claiming I'm advocating starvation of infants. What I'm advocating is a sensible, careful approach to feeding young children, with parents as conscious of the dangers of overfeeding as they are of underfeeding. This is a time when parental knowledge of diet and nutrition is crucial, and I hope you will keep yourselves well-informed when it is time for you to have children.

The second critical period in which you can accumulate fat cells at a very rapid pace is during adolescence, from ages 10 to 16. This is the period that many of you are in or are approaching—and it is part of the focus of this book—a time when you must depend on your family for their help, but must also learn to help yourself, to monitor your own diet, and to think about and prevent an increase in fat cells.

There are two more periods in the female lifetime when it is easier to create more fat cells. One is during pregnancy and the other is while taking the birth control pill. Both of these are periods of high hormonal stimulation. During the nine months of pregnancy, the whole body seems to go into overtime to produce fat, used for the nourishment of the baby.

And in the overweight female, the birth control pill makes it 10 percent easier to gain weight. Therefore, if and when you start taking birth control pills, it will be necessary to cut back 10 percent in your food intake, just to maintain your weight. Remember, birth control pills or pills of similar composition are sometimes also given for relief of severe menstrual cramps and for some forms of acne that won't respond to usual methods of treatment.

During other periods of your life you may gain smaller amounts of weight if you overeat, merely overstuffing existing fat cells, and you can lose that weight relatively easily by decreasing your food intake. But once you create *new* fat cells, you'll never lose them—they just get bigger or smaller.

3

Why Do People Get Fat?

Every textbook on nutrition states that people get fat by taking in more calories than they expend or, to put it simply, by eating too much and exercising too little.

But all around us we see exceptions to this rule. Think of all the people that you know who can eat enormous quantities of food and never gain an ounce. (And their most strenuous activity is talking on the telephone!)

On the other hand, some of us play tennis, run, haven't dared to eat dessert in a month, and still gain weight.

Clearly, not everyone gets fat. Why? Food is certainly available, legal, safe, delicious—why doesn't everyone have double chins and potbellies? The answer, of course, is that it's not as simple as eating too much and exercising too little.

Overweight is a complex and poorly-understood condition that is caused by several factors. These include:

Heredity
Environment
Emotions
Choice of Foods

Heredity

Skinny people like to think that you get fat because you have no "will power." This implies that you are so weak that by comparison they are pillars of physical and mental strength. That's not true; they are thin because they are born that way, not because they're superior beings.

If one of your parents is overweight, there's a 40 percent chance that you will be, too. If both parents are overweight, your chances jump to 80 percent. If neither parent has a weight problem, you have a 10 percent chance of developing one; there may be a fat gene somewhere in your family tree.

Some "experts" claim that these odds exist because fat parents feed their children the same fattening things that they eat. Environment, they say, is the most important cause of overweight. I violently disagree with this theory because it doesn't explain why in a family of three children with a fat mother, only one or two of the children may be fat. The mother clearly presents the same food to all three; why does only one gain weight?

A recent Canadian study followed the growth of 200 adopted children and found that the child's body type most often resembled the *natural* parents, not the adopted ones. Therefore, if you haven't inherited the tendency to be overweight, chances are you will never be extremely fat, no matter what your environment is like.

Thin people (mostly men) often ask me how to gain weight. I have tried to help them, but no matter how many calories some of them eat, they barely gain a pound. The thin people are not necessarily more active or more nervous than the overweight ones; they seem to have an inefficient fat-storing mechanism in their bodies.

In one study, thin male volunteers were fed 8,000 calories a day in an attempt to "fatten them up." At the end of 6 months, each man gained 28 to 30 pounds. After scientists deducted the amount of calories burned through exercise, they estimated that each man should have gained 240 pounds!

I think that people who can't gain weight are very lucky, and I envy them, but they constantly worry about how bad they look.

Body Build

There are three basic types of inherited body builds: the *ectomorph*, the *mesomorph*, and the *endomorph*.

The ectomorph is the tall, slender body type with long fingers. This person rarely has a weight problem.

The mesomorph is the jock type, more frequently a male because this build requires a substantial amount of muscle mass.

Mesomorphs can look heavy, and most weigh more than normal, but this weight is muscle, not fat. Mesomorphs can have a weight problem but it usually comes when they have been slowed down by injury or illness and keep eating as if they were active. However, once they assume normal activity, their appetites return to normal and so does their weight.

The build that I see most often in my office is the endomorph. Endomorph is the *soft, rounded, stocky, padded, short-pudgy-fingered, lateral build* that spells trouble. The shorter the endomorph, the less calories he/she seems to require to gain or maintain weight. I have seen endomorphs gain weight on 1,500 calories per day and have to decrease their daily food intake to 700 calories to lose weight.

Appetite

Appetites are born, not made. Some people are born with large appetites, other are satisfied by smaller quantities of food. Many of the people who find it difficult to lose weight have larger than normal appetites, despite their claims that they don't eat a lot. A large appetite can get larger or smaller, depending on the food presented, but normal appetites tend to stay constant.

What makes some people eat more food than others? Not true hunger, because hunger is a physical sign and should have a beginning and an end. What seems to make overweights want more to eat is their heightened sensitivity to the sight, smell, and taste of food. They are "food suggestible," which means that they can usually be prevailed upon to taste something that they do not necessarily want. However, once they sample something sugary, it triggers an urge to eat more sugar. They eat and can't stop eating until they are physically sick. In a very short time they can take in an enormous amount of calories.

Everyone has this sugar-triggering mechanism, but in people of normal weight that trigger is set at a much higher level. In other words, if a normal person ate 10 pieces of candy, he could probably set off this mechanism, but it would be unusual for him to eat this much in the first place. With the overweight teen-age girl, it takes only two pieces of candy, and she eats that much all the time. This leads to those wild "binges" that are responsible for much of her excess weight.

Metabolic Imbalance

Most mothers want to believe that their overweight daughters have inherited a metabolic or glandular problem, specifically in the production of thyroid.

The thyroid gland sits at the base of the neck and secretes a hormone that plays an important role in the breakdown of fat. "Would you check my daughter's thyroid?" is a question I hear many times a week in my office. And I always comply, even though 99 percent of the test results are normal.

It's possible that there is something wrong with your thyroid gland if you have more difficulty losing weight than most people. Either it is not putting out enough thyroid hormone (in which case it is under- or hypoactive) or there is something wrong with the thyroid that it is producing.

Since I rarely find abnormally low levels of thyroid in blood tests of overweight girls, I sometimes reason that the thyroid present in their bodies is not doing its job. In these cases I prescribe additional thyroid.

Why do mothers and daughters keep looking to thyroid as an answer to their weight problems? Because everyone would like to think that there is a physical reason for their obesity. Frequently there is, but thyroid alone won't solve the problems. Caloric intake will still have to be cut drastically.

The second metabolic irregularity in obese teen-agers is their inability to handle carbohydrates. (This gets worse with age.) They seen unable to convert sugar and some starches into energy as efficiently as they should. They burn 1,000 calories of carbohydrates differently—and with greater difficulty—than 1,000 calories of protein. This could be because breaking down certain foods raises the basal metabolic rate (BMR, the oxygen intake and carbon dioxide released in a resting state), causing an added expenditure of energy.

Some scientists think that if these metabolic imbalances do exist, they have been *caused* by excess weight. In other words, there were no metabolic defects until the person became obese. I think that both arguments have their merit. Some imbalance does exist at birth, but the accumulation of more and more fat makes the problem much more severe. For example, when a very heavy female (250 to 300 pounds) begins to diet, her initial weight loss is difficult and slow. As her weight drops closer to normal levels, her body chemistry changes, and weight loss becomes easier.

Exercise Tolerance

I would change the old saying, "You can lead a horse to water, but you can't make him drink," to "You can lead an overweight to the track, but you can't make her run." I constantly battle my overweight patients to get them to move, but they just don't want to budge. Their mothers tell me that as babies these girls always preferred sitting to running around, and as young children they preferred tea parties and tid-dlywinks to kickball or rope-jumping. As teen-agers, they do less spontaneous exercise than any other age group.

But it's wishful thinking to say, "I'll be more active when I lose weight," because it's not the weight that's slowing you down. Endo-morphs have naturally low energy levels, which will be present whether they are fat or thin. They can discipline themselves to be active (we will discuss how this can be done later), but they will never have the spontaneous "get-up-and-go" of their thin sisters.

If you are overweight and decide to begin an exercise program, you may come across a chart like this:

Activity	Calories burned per minute	Activity	Calories burned per minute
Resting in bed	1	Ping-Pong	5
Standing	2	Swimming	8
Walking, indoors	3	Golfing	5
Walking up stairs	14	Tennis	7
Standing, showering	4	Bowling*	5
Making beds	5	Running	10
Mopping floors	5	Dancing	5
Peeling vegetables	3	Horseback riding	3
Shoveling	7	Cycling	8
Basketball	9		

Looks good doesn't it? But as a female, especially an overweight female, you don't burn calories like this. These calorie charts were

*A friend once described bowling as "the only sport in which you gain weight," because it's so natural to chomp on candy bars and potato chips between balls, and then to go for a pizza.

made for men whose body temperatures are much higher and whose muscle burns more calories than your soft tissue. I'm not trying to discourage you from exercising—just don't depend on it too heavily for weight loss. Cut those calorie-burning charts in half to get a more realistic picture of the way your body produces energy.

To sum up what I have said here, there are certain inherited characteristics that give you the potential to be fat: the ability to create too many fat cells; an endomorphic build with the emphasis on fat rather than muscle; an increased appetite with a sensitive triggering mechanism for sweets; possible hormonal or metabolic imbalances; a difficulty in converting carbohydrates to energy; and an innate laziness and poor level of energy expenditure. So much for "eating too much and exercising too little."

Environment

I believe that heredity plays the most important role in becoming and staying fat. I'm not saying that environment isn't important, but I feel that no matter how bad your environment—with respect to food, family relations, and so on—you won't get *very* fat if you haven't inherited the tendency.

However, a potentially fat child born into an environment that encourages light feeding, lots of exercise, and few high-calorie snacks can expect to go through life less fat than her less fortunate counterpart, who eats huge, high-calorie meals and exercises very little. The family is the key to controlling your weight up to a certain age. And if your family uses food as a reward, as love, and as a bribe, you will be fatter at a younger age.

Stress within the family is a very common reason for diet failure. Many teen-agers tell me that it is almost impossible to diet in a home where:

1. there are frequent arguments between parents
2. one parent is an alcoholic

Food in those situations seems to supply a great deal of comfort and makes going home bearable.

Some families are food-oriented. Refrigerators are stuffed with delicious leftovers; cabinets are filled with junk foods; and so much food is served at supper that the table nearly collapses under the weight. Then there are the food rituals: baking cookies for Christmas, canning fruit in July, and baking bread every Sunday. This kind of environment is a nightmare for the teen-ager trying to diet.

Emotions

Emotions play a large role in making and keeping teen-agers fat. It's not the emotions themselves, you understand, but the behavior that the emotions trigger. Many women ask, "Can nerves make you fat?" I reply, "Only if you overeat when you're nervous."

Many psychiatrists claim that overeating is a sign of deep emotional problems. The four problems to which they often allude are:

1. use of food as a substitute for love
2. use of food to discourage the opposite sex
3. use of food to spite someone
4. food = mood

I think that we all have a mental picture of the poor lonely fat girl nobody loves, stuffing cake into her mouth on a Saturday night, while her girl friends are out partying. Although this girl still exists, she is not as common as she used to be. Many overweight girls have friends, go to lots of parties, and even date.

The second reason for emotional eating might be more valid. There is something protective about being overweight and not dating as much (or at all). There are no decisions to make about who to kiss and who not to kiss, no advances to fight off, no temptations. Many teen-agers tell me, quite honestly, that they're glad they're not popular with boys. "I would worry all night about what would happen at the end of the evening," one of them confided. Food is a comfortable alternative to sex.

A new theory about emotional overeating is that some women stay overweight to appear "substantial" and to call attention to themselves. I thought that this was totally preposterous until I visited one of my son's favorite teachers, shortly after the publication of my first book. "What makes you think everyone wants to be thin?" she demanded. "I like being big. It gives me a sense of power. It makes people turn around and look at me." On another occasion, a parent explained to me how her child got fat. "We moved to a neighborhood with a tough school," she said, "and I noticed Robin gaining weight. 'That's so I can protect myself,' she told me. 'Nobody will dare pick on me.'" Some women may enjoy feeling tough and powerful, perhaps as a protest against the concept of a "weaker" sex.

The third reason for emotional overeating is overemphasized, but nonetheless frequently used. When children learn how concerned parents are over their intake of food, they also learn they can use it as a weapon, a threat, or a protest. *Refusing* to eat becomes the ultimate act of defiance, but hunger is uncomfortable and most children give in after a short time. The overweight youngster quickly learns to eat too much—it's not only an act of defiance, but it's much more pleasant. How else can you please yourself and yet irritate the people who care for you?

Finally, the most important emotional reason for eating is the idea that mood = food. Moods like boredom, frustration, anger, and nervousness create tension, and often people eat to relieve this tension. Pretty soon it becomes automatic: "I'm bored, so I'll eat"; "I'm angry, so I'll eat." Some people think that they can escape from their problems by eating, and while they eat they do often forget what's bothering them. When they finish, however, the problems come back, except they feel even worse because they've eaten so much.

Choice of Foods

Eating junk has become a national pastime. Think of all those bold, sugary tastes packaged in little cellophane bags for quick, effortless grabbing. This is a time of fast food, junk food, and sugar-sugar-everywhere, and every mouthful is a caloric disaster.

If you are going to eat a lot of food with refined sugar and flour, you're going to lose track of the number of calories going into your mouth. For example, a very small bag of my favorite cheese twists is 285 calories. I could eat five bags—easily. When food was simple and plain, we ate to satisfy hunger. Now we eat to excite the taste buds and treat the tummy. Is it surprising that today's world gets rounder and rounder?

4

Thinking You Are Overweight

Most of the people who read this book will be either teen-agers who have a weight problem or their parents. But there are many girls without weight problems who will be quite interested in these pages— normal girls who *think* they are overweight.

What makes normal girls fear they are overweight? Usually they are daughters of mothers who are always dieting and talking about their bodies. Daughters who want to get recognition from their mothers frequently try to identify with them by imitating their weight preoccupations. In this way, daughters and mothers become closer, or so they think. Actually, this kind of role modeling is common and not particularly unhealthy, as long as both mother and daughter realize that they are playing a kind of game.

The second reason is that photographic or fashion modeling is coming closer and closer to teen-age levels. Models used to be mainly adult females, but since the tremendous upsurge of teen magazines, the teen model has come into her own.

Interestingly enough, the teen model is usually a good 10 to 20 pounds heavier than her adult replica, almost as if Madison Avenue (the people who dream up the ads) is fearful of starving the younger female, waiting instead until she reaches the age of emancipation (18) before setting such rigid standards on her body.

The third reason for preoccupation with weight is the emergence of sports for females. Once girls used their bodies only for exhibiting themselves in beauty contests. Now women's bodies have become more functional, and in certain areas leanness is a necessity.

Coaches tell us that the leaner the female swimmer is, the faster she goes. Even a slight amount of excess weight on dancers seems to drive ballet masters up the wall. I have seen young girls turned into blithering idiots by dance instructors who were absolutely hysterical over weight gains of 2 to 3 pounds. With this kind of tension, it's no surprise that some girls are so uptight.

Another normal reason for feeling that you're overweight when you're not is the physical transition from little girl to young woman. This involves the distribution of fat into hips, upper legs, and breasts. A girl who has been long and lean and virtually without curves may look down one day and see an increase in body proportions. She naturally assumes she is getting fatter. Teen-age girls constantly pinch the tops of their legs, demanding that everybody "look at all that fat." This often starts a lifetime of trying to get rid of normal fat distribution that is very much a part of being a female.

The above are normal reasons for worrying about weight. These girls will diet frequently but they will rarely harm their bodies in any way. Most of them will give up when they see how difficult it is to keep as lean as they want. Sometimes dieting just gives them something to talk about. They want to attract attention and to hear people say, "Oh, you don't need to diet at all. You have a beautiful figure." Many girls enjoy this sort of gratification and constantly repeat their act.

Finally, we come to the abnormal person with a weight preoccupation.

Anorexia Nervosa

"I see a lot of skinny people. I used to know a girl in sixth grade and we used to weigh the same. I look at her now and I don't think she ate. She made herself not eat and now I'd say she weighs about 80 or 90 pounds and it's gross. Her bones are sticking out everywhere. Her nose is always red and she always has a coat on and it's gross, you know? I'd rather be overweight than like that. I don't know how well she eats, but everyone says she should go to a doctor and it's gross. Just as gross as being overweight."

A Classmate

Tracey—A Case History

Tracey twiddled a little flap of skin beneath her chin and wondered why she'd never had a boyfriend. She had been staring into the mirror for so long that her eyes ached, but she didn't feel like studying, and her mother wouldn't let her go out in the rain.

Why, Tracey thought, don't boys find me attractive? She used to think she had beautiful dark eyes, which were almost as dark as her hair. She was 5 feet 5 inches tall, as tall as her mother, and taller than her older sister. Tracey wished she had a brother—then she could ask him what was wrong with the way she looked.

Or even a father. She didn't remember him very well, and her mother wouldn't permit her to mention him. Tracey was only 5 years old when he left. It was not a good time.

> Tracey was 15 years old, weighed 135 pounds, and was 5 feet 5 inches tall. She was raised, along with her older sister, by a divorced mother in a resort area of Miami. Her mother was extremely strict and did not allow Tracey or her sister to date, even in high school.
>
> Tracey's mother kept her so inhibited that she appeared cold and withdrawn to any boy she met. That was okay with the boys—Tracey's school had a female to male ratio of 3 to 1. Shy, dark-haired Tracey did not attract attention.
>
> "I decided it was because I was too fat," explained Tracey later. "I had to lose weight, and I had to lose it quickly."
>
> *December 1.* Tracey puts herself on a very rigid diet of 800 calories per day.
>
> *January 3.* Tracey returns to classes after Christmas break. She weighs 117 pounds. Her social life does not change. "I spend hours looking at myself in the mirror. Everything else was okay. I was just too fat."
>
> *January 9.* Tracey resumes her diet. This time she exercises an hour a day—calisthenics and jogging.
>
> *February 1.* Tracey weighs 104 pounds. Classmates notice this strange, dark-haired girl getting thinner and thinner. Instead of asking for dates, the boys keep as far away as possible.
>
> *February 5.* Tracey's mother becomes frantic over her daughter's refusal to eat. She takes her daughter to the family doctor. There, Tracey carefully explains her problems with the opposite sex. The doctor orders her to eat. She says she'll think about it.
>
> *February 14.* Tracey turns 16. Her periods are regular. She has a slight breast development, but few friends and no birthday party.

February 20. Tracey weighs 96 pounds. Her mother takes her back to the family doctor, who, alarmed, refers them to a psychiatrist.

February 22. Tracey begins psychotherapy. Again, she calmly explains her problem, and even jokes with the doctor.

March 25. Tracey weighs 80 pounds. She is so starved she can barely walk. Her grades have dropped sharply. She tells her mother she looks fine and enjoys being slender. "What's the fuss about?" she asks.

March 27. Tracey is admitted to a psychiatric hospital. Doctors fear she will die from lack of nutrition and transfer her to a general hospital. There, a tube is put in her nose and down her throat, feeding her a liquid mixture to make her gain weight.

April 10. Tracey is transferred to a psychiatric hospital. She weighs 100 pounds and is out of danger. She appears to be a charming, outgoing, sophisticated young lady. No one can convince her there was anything wrong with her behavior. The doctors tell her that if she doesn't eat, she will be fed again through tubes. She begins to eat normally.

April 30. Tracey is discharged from the psychiatric hospital. She has a great deal more insight into her personality problems, but no idea why she hadn't been able to stop starving herself.

Do you think Tracey was a normal girl who just got carried away with her diet?

No. Tracey had anorexia nervosa (which means a loss of appetite originating in the nervous system), a psychiatric illness.

Anorexia nervosa has had a lot of press in the past few years, though it is still an unusual disease. One publication called it "The 'die' in dieting," which implies it is a potential hazard for anyone who takes dieting too seriously.

I don't agree. Normal dieters do not become anorexic. This particular mental disease seems to afflict primarily white, middle-class, teen-age females (there are some males, but this is rare) and leads to loss of appetite to the point of starvation, stopping of menstrual periods, and, sometimes, death.

Anorexia is *abnormal* behavior, not normal behavior gone haywire. Although psychiatrists blame the disease on domineering mothers with high expectations or anorexics' use of food as a weapon to strike back at their families (the same reason, they say, for overeating), I don't think environment is the sole problem. (Tracey's sister was perfectly normal.)

It is a *basic individual personality problem* that leads anorexics past dieting and into more destructive behavior. The relationship between dieting and anorexia seems to me as imperfect as the relationship between smoking marijuana and shooting heroin. One *may* lead to the other, but this is the exception rather than the rule.

Anorexia seems to be more common during the first or second year of college than in high school, probably because competition and stress are greater, and it is a major period of adjustment for girls.

I believe that anorexia is a symptom of a more severe psychiatric illness, and it doesn't happen without a lot of warnings. Often we read in the newspaper that some adult or adolescent has starved herself to death, frequently in the presence of many people, people who see what's going on but fail to act.

Anorexics need psychiatric care, but first they must be prevented from starving themselves. If you have friends who are behaving this way, I implore you to tell somebody who will help. If their parents won't pay attention, talk to a teacher or school counselor. Anorexics lack the ability to halt their starvation—that's part of their sickness. They need somebody to halt it *for* them.

For a while, the results of treatment of anorexics were very depressing, with a large percentage of deaths. Lately, more behavioral approaches have been found to work.

You have to realize that nobody reasons with anorexics! They are *deluded* by the thought that they are fat. I was amazed when I heard how one psychiatrist treated anorexic patients. He brought a mirror into his office and made them look into it and said, "Look, you're much too thin." This makes absolutely no impression on these girls. At this state, they want to be thin and are never satisfied with the degree of thinness.

The new approach is simply to tell them, "Look, if you don't eat, we are going to put a tube up your nose and down your throat." Therapists don't wait long to do this, either. Unless they see a progressive weight gain, they hospitalize the patient and proceed to "refeed." There are excellent, well-balanced liquid mixtures now, perfectly suited to the anorexic's needs.

Anorexic patients are really quite vain and hate to see tubes sticking out of their noses. They don't enjoy the feeling of tubes going down their throats, either. Many times they will say, "I'd rather eat than be tube-fed." Also, their hospital privileges depend on the amount of weight that they gain. Often, they are not allowed to call home or see parents until there is a steady, progressive weight gain, and if there is any backsliding, privileges are taken away. They are *re-taught* to eat minimum portions of food and *reprogrammed* until they are eating normally.

Psychotherapy still plays a role in trying to get the anorexic to understand the facet in their personality that made them ill. But psychotherapy has only been of value when combined with behavioral retraining.

To repeat, anorexia nervosa is a special condition, the exception, not the rule. It will not be brought on by enthusiastic dieting.

It is interesting to compare personality features of the normal dieter (the true overweight) to the anorexic.

Anorexic	*Normal Dieter*
1. Usually only mildly overweight, if overweight at all.	1. Mild to severe overweight.
2. Extremely sensitive about any remarks made about weight.	2. Varies from being slightly sensitive to taking it with a grain of salt.
3. Allows seemingly minor fluctuations in weight to get in the way of doing things and going places.	3. Usually will go places if she can find something to wear. Goes to the beach, but doesn't wear a bathing suit.
4. Feels the reasons people don't like her is connected to her weight.	4. Feels her weight does not influence the way people feel about her, especially the other girls.
5. Perfectionist, extremely orderly.	5. Ranges from being somewhat neat to being a slob.
6. Expresses much concern for order.	6. Casual about orderliness. Somewhat haphazard about lifestyle and appearance.
7. Refuses to eat or avoids food.	7. Relishes every 'mouthful. Enjoys looking at food; easily tempted.
8. Exercises and moves constantly, sometimes at a frantic pace.	8. Must beg to get any coordinated exercise. Difficult to get moving.
9. Loves dieting and enjoys being very thin. Preoccupied with weight.	9. Hates dieting. Feels angry at the world for having to diet.
10. Goes into food rituals. Cuts things into little pieces; moves things around the plate and pretends she is eating. Hoards food instead of eating.	10. Food rituals are a bore. Would rather gulp down food. Doesn't hoard anything because she eats it before she can hoard it. Only takes time eating and cutting food methodically if she is on a behavior modification program.
11. Appetite seems gone.	11. Appetite just checked and can emerge at full force any time.
12. Usually wants to go very far below desired weight, and does.	12. Usually wants to go below desired weight but stops slightly higher.
13. Will vomit and take laxatives to feel thin.	13. Rarely vomits unless she is sick. Often interprets gagging as vomiting. Bowel movements are excellent, and she would not think of taking a laxative.
14. Periods will stop.	14. Periods might become irregular or change in character as normal weight is approached, but generally remain the same.
15. The more she looks like a cadaver, the more pleased she will be with herself.	15. If she looks too thin, she will get worried that she might be sick.

5

Food and Nutrition

I was always bored by the way my old high-school teachers taught nutrition—long, dry explanations of energy, calories, proteins, carbo-hydrates, and fats.

That's essentially what I want to talk about, but the field of nutrition has changed radically in the last decade, and it's now one of the most exciting and important frontiers in all of preventive medicine. It still involves the study of over-nutrition (obesity) and under-nutrition (starvation), but scientists have begun to discover the effect of the food we eat on our general health, life span, ability to fight off illness and infection, and even to endure stress.

First, the basics:

Food is composed of *nutrients*, which are grouped into five categories: protein; carbohydrates; fats (macronutrients); and vitamins and minerals (micronutrients). Food serves as fuel for energy, which produces work. Because all work takes the form of heat production, energy can be measured in terms of heat. To simplify, *energy leads to work; work leads to heat; heat is measured in calories.* The calorie concept is rather dull, but in dieting it's important.

How are calories measured? A weighed amount of food is placed in a calorimeter (called a "bomb" because of its shape), and the instrument is immersed in water. The food is ignited and burned, and the temperature increase of the surrounding water indicates the heat given off by the burning of food. That heat is measured by the calorie, which is the amount of heat required to raise 1 kilogram of water 1 degree centigrade. Actually, the correct nutrient measurement is a kilocalorie, which is 1,000 calories.

A piece of Boston cream pie contains 350 calories that are activated only when the pie is eaten and digested. Therefore, where food is concerned, the calorie is the potential of a substance to produce energy. Food for thought: If that piece of cake remains in the refrigerator, will it still have 350 calories?

I have trouble believing in the concept of the calorie. It assumes that the body is a *perfect machine* like the "bomb," one that converts food to energy at 100 percent efficiency. But the overweight female is not a perfect machine.

Let's talk about how nutrition directly affects your life. The following statements are extremely important for you to consider:

1. *McGovern Report.* Six of the ten major killer diseases are related to diet. They are heart disease, obesity, diabetes, hypertension, cancer, and cerebrovascular disease.
2. *A Headline.* Surveys indicate that teen-age girls consume the least nutritious foods of any age or sex group. Old enough to choose their food, they choose candy bars far too often.
3. *A Headline.* Poor choices and frantic dieting give teen-age girls "roller coaster" eating habits.

McGovern Report: Nutrition is the science of food and its relationship to health. Not too long ago poor health was defined as being too fat or too skinny. But things have changed. In 1978, the study *The Dietary Goals for the United States* was released by the Senate Nutrition Subcommittee, which was chaired by Senator George McGovern. This document was a breakthrough because it was the first attempt by a government agency to suggest a national policy on nutrition.

A good understanding of current nutrition can be achieved if we examine the seven McGovern goals more closely. We will discuss each one in terms of *what it means, what you should know about the general subject* (that the study may not tell you), *what to do about it*, and *words that you should remember.*

Goal 1

To avoid overweight consume energy (calories) only as it is expended. If overweight, decrease energy intake and increase energy expenditure.

This means: If you are overweight, eat less and exercise more.

The average, moderately active teen-age female needs 2,100 to 2,400 calories daily, depending on her height and weight. She burns around a calorie per minute just by breathing, and considerably more by moving. Her body requires 10 to 15 calories for every pound of body weight.

A pound of fat is 3,500 calories. A decrease in daily caloric intake of 500 calories or an increase in daily energy output of 500 calories, *while keeping caloric intake the same*, will lead to a loss of one pound per week (7 × 500 = 3500).

What you should know:

1. Goal 1 doesn't always work. Sometimes you are eating very little, exercising a great deal, and you're still not losing weight—another example of the human body as an imperfect machine.
2. Maintenance level is often set too high for teen-age females because it does not take into account those girls who are not active or those girls with an inherited tendency to be overweight.

Words you should know:

1. *Calorie.* A unit to measure the heat produced as energy and released while the body performs work. The unit of measure is the *large calorie* or *kilocalorie* which is equal to 1,000 small calories. A kilocalorie is the amount of heat required to raise one kilogram of water one degree centigrade.
2. *Energy.* That force of power that enables the body to carry on life-sustaining activities.
3. *Basal Metabolic Rate (BMR).* The amount of energy needed by your body for maintenance of life when you are at rest. Your BMR is the number of calories you burn just by breathing.

Goal 2

Increase comsumption of complex carbohydrates and "naturally-occurring sugars" from 28 percent of energy intake to 48 percent of energy intake.

This means: Eat more starch and natural sugar. Natural sugar refers to the sugars found in fruits and vegetables, *not* the refined sugars of sweets.

Carbohydrates (starches and sugars) provide the most available, economical source of energy for the human body and supply four calories of energy per gram.

Chemically, carbohydrates are made up of carbon, hydrogen, and oxygen. The simplest carbohydrate is called sugar. Glucose is the most important sugar in the body. A complex carbohydrate is made up of many chains of simple sugars. Starch is the most significant complex carbohydrate and makes up over 50 percent of our carbohydrate intake.

In order to fulfill Goal 2, try to include daily servings of leafy green or yellow vegetables, all fruits, potatoes, breads, and cereals. Use more rice and bean products. The last five items represent starch.

What you should know: In the last few years, "carbohydrate" has become a dirty word for dieters. With the advent of the popular high-protein, low-carbohydrate diets, the implication has been that carbohydrates, or sugars and starches, make people fat. The dissenters argue that 500 calories of protein equal 500 calories of carbohydrate equals 500 calories of fat. They say it is ridiculous to take carbohydrates out of a diet, because:

1. the body needs a balanced diet,
2. carbohydrate is the preferred energy source for the brain and muscle, and
3. carbohydrate is available and economical.

Those of us who work in dieting and particularly those of us who have worked with females have observed that diets high in carbohydrates, but normal in calories, do the following things:

1. stimulate appetite
2. promote fluid retention
3. slow down weight loss
4. cause fatigue

Interestingly enough, the first and last of these observations suggest that carbohydrates do the exact opposite of what they are supposed to do: they do not satisfy appetite or increase energy. Obviously, the overweight female body does not play by the rules of normal food breakdown.

If carbohydrate is truly preferred brain and muscle food, cutting down on it won't devastate your intelligence or your strength—it is available in acceptable quantities from other foods, such as vegetables. But some recent data suggests that *fat* might be the preferred source of brain energy.

There's only one way for you to judge whether a low-low-carbohydrate diet is right for you: try it for one week. Eat only meat, fish, eggs, cheese, lettuce, cucumbers, grapefruit, and diet gelatin desserts. Remember to take a multivitamin pill every day. See how you feel. If you lose weight, feel good, think better, and have more pep, then you're sensitive to carbohydrates. They should be kept at a minimum in dieting and at a low-to-moderate level in maintaining your weight.

Goal 3

Reduce consumption of refined and processed sugar by about 45 percent to account for about 10 percent of total energy intake.

This means: Stop eating sugar.

Use as little sugar as possible in cooking. Take the sugar bowl off the table. Read labels and avoid foods that have sugar high on the list of ingredients.

We have been victims of the philosophy, "If a little bit tastes good, a lot must taste better." Sugar is everywhere, in everything—even where we don't expect it.

One nutritionist suggests that our love of sugar is acquired, not natural. I disagree. Certain tribal children were brought to the United States at the age of 6 and for the first time in their lives tasted candy. They loved it although they had never tasted it before. Love of sweetness is built into out systems: primitive man used the taste of sweetness to differentiate safe food from poisonous food; and man's first food, milk, contains large amounts of lactose, a milk sugar.

What you should know:

1. Nothing makes you fatter quicker than refined sugar.
2. The first taste of sugar triggers the appetites of most overweight females.
3. Refined sugar gives you empty calories and a pleasant taste, but isn't even filling. It is far better to eat carbohydrates with higher nutritional value, such as the starches and natural sugars.

Words you should know:

1. *Sugar.* A carbohydrate that may have a "single" chemical chain (monosaccharide) or a "double" chemical chain (disaccharide). The body rapidly oxidizes sugars to yield carbon dioxide and water; this process is a major source of body heat and energy.

2. *Monosaccharide.* The simplest form of carbohydrate, made up of carbon, hydrogen, and oxygen, often called a "simple sugar."
3. *Glucose.* The most common sugar, which is moderately sweet. In human metabolism all other types of sugar are converted into glucose, which circulates in the bloodstream and is oxidized to give energy.
4. *Fructose.* A simple sugar that is found in fruits and honey. Fructose accounts for the sweetest of the simple sugars and is converted to glucose for energy.
5. *Disaccharide.* A sugar made up of two monosaccharides. The three main disaccharides are sucrose (common table sugar), lactose (the sugar in milk), and maltose (found in malt products).
6. *Lactose.* A disaccharide that is the sugar in milk. It is formed in the body from glucose to supply the carbohydrate component of milk during lactation. It is the least sweet of the disaccharides, about one-sixth as sweet as sucrose.
7. *Polysaccharide.* A carbohydrate that is even more complex than complex sugars. Starch is the most significant polysaccharide in human nutrition.

Goal 4

Reduce overall fat consumption from approximately 40 percent to about 30 percent of energy intake.

This means: Cut down on fat.

Plan some meals with vegetable proteins. Use anything low-fat. Boil (yes, I said boil), meat. Decrease consumption of animal fat by eating more fish and poultry.

Fat is a nutrient that supplies 9 calories per gram or 100 calories per tablespoon—over twice as much energy as carbohydrates. The building blocks of fat are fatty acids. Fat is also necessary for the absorption of vitamins A, D, E, and K and serves as protection for organs and nerves. Fat is usually easy to recognize since it's greasy and oily to the touch. Fats include butter, mayonnaise, egg yolk, avocado, and nuts.

What you should know:

1. Diets low in fat lead to dry skin—which is peculiar because you are breaking down so much body fat.
2. Fat is deceptive. If you order a salad with 50 calories, you may unwittingly douse it with 300 calories of salad dressing. If you get a cooked vegetable that has 30 calories you might find there are 150 calories of butter in it. If you are not losing weight, beware of the "hidden 100" (100 calories of fat in everything you think is cooked dry).

Words you should know:

1. *Lipids.* The group name for fats. The lipids include fats, oils, waxes, and related compounds.
2. *Saturated Fat.* A fatty acid is said to be saturated if all available chemical bonds of its carbon chain are filled with hydrogen. Fats of animal sources are more saturated than those of vegetable sources.
3. *Unsaturated Fat.* If one of the available chemical bonds of the fatty acid's carbon chain is unfilled, it is a monounsaturated fatty acid. If two or more bonds remain unfilled, it is a polyunsaturated fatty acid. Fats of plant sources are more unsaturated than fats of animal sources.
5. *Lipoprotein.* Compounds of fat with protein. The basic function of the lipoproteins is to transport cholesterol and triglycerides in the bloodstream. Low Density Lipoproteins (LDL) carry the cholesterol that lodges in the walls of the arteries, promoting arteriosclerosis. The High Density Lipoproteins (HDL) act to remove cholesterol and, therefore, may protect the arteries.
6. *Ketosis.* High level of unburned fatty acids in body, caused by incomplete burning of fat as a fuel. Ketosis is a characteristic of high-protein, low-carbohydrate diets. The ketons are acids, and their accumulation upsets the normal pH in the body. This tends to depress the appetite.

     You become ketotic after a sustained period of starvation (for example, when you get up in the morning after sleeping 8 hours). At that point you start to break down fat for energy, but do not have any carbohydrate available to complete the burning process.

Goal 5

Reduce saturated fat consumption to account for about 10 percent of total energy intake and balance that with polyunsaturated and monounsaturated fats, which should account for about 10 percent of energy intake each.

This means: Twenty percent of your diet will be fat. Eat more fat that is liquid at room temperature (such as corn oil and safflower oil). These are unsaturated fats.

Fats from animal sources that are solid at room temperature (such as meat and butter) are saturated.

What you should know: Saturated fat probably has more effect on the development of heart disease and hardening of the arteries than unsaturated fat. About two thirds of the fat eaten by Americans is saturated. The remaining third is unsaturated. Goal 5 is trying to reverse that ratio. There is evidence that the substitution of unsaturated for saturated fat lessens the risk of heart disease.

Goal 6

Reduce cholesterol consumption to about 300 milligrams a day.

This means: What it says.

Arteriosclerosis causes heart disease. Fatty degeneration and thickening occur on the inside walls of the coronary arteries, forming *plaques* that narrow the diameter of the vessel and make blood flow slowly. This, in turn, can lead to blood clots and the eventual closing off of the involved artery. When this artery is closed off, the heart is deprived of vital oxygen, and a heart attack may occur.

Cholesterol is a fatty compound that is needed to form certain hormones. It is found in egg yolk, organ meat (for example, kidney and liver), and shrimp, and it is also manufactured in the body. The problem is that it is the major component of those fatty plaques that block the coronary artery.

What you should know:

1. Heart disease before menopause is not a major problem in females. But the number of deaths due to coronary artery disease after menopause (around age 65) equals that of males.
2. The body probably manufactures more cholesterol on its own than you ingest. Therefore, a decrease in your cholesterol intake does not necessarily mean that there will be a dramatic drop in your blood cholesterol level.
3. Many individuals tolerate cholesterol well. Some show no response to changes in cholesterol intake. Certain volunteers were fed 3 eggs a day along with other high cholesterol foods, with very little change in their serum cholesterol. The relationship between cholesterol and heart disease is not as clear-cut as many people would have us believe.

   A large egg alone contains about 250 milligrams of cholesterol.
4. Teen-age females who have normal levels of cholesterol should be advised that eggs are excellent food. If you like them, you should eat them without hesitation.

Goal 7

Limit the intake of sodium by reducing the intake of salt to about five grams per day.

This means: The average daily amount of sodium in the American diet is ten grams of table salt. You should: (1) take the salt shaker off the table and (2) watch out for canned or dried soups and salad dressings that are high in salt.

What you should know:

1. This goal was set up because salt was found to cause some types of high blood pressure (hypertension). Salt has no effect on blood pressure unless there is a preexisting tendency to be hypertensive.
2. The salt goal is the most unacceptable as far as the normal dieting female teen-ager is concerned. The chances that too much salt will give her high blood pressure are remote. Sixty percent of my obese *adult* female patients are hypertensive solely on the basis of their weight. There is no question that excess weight leads to hypertension in females, but they can obtain normal blood pressures through small weight losses without decreasing salt. The reduction of *weight, not salt* is an important factor in female hypertension.
3. Reduction of salt in the normal female dieter is sometimes useful for the prevention of fluid retention. Decrease salt the week before your period, and you won't feel as bloated or gain as much weight.

Well, after discussing the United States government's dietary goals, I now offer my opinion: I think they should be taken with a grain of salt (no pun intended). I don't think that any single dietary recommendation is appropriate for all segments of our population. The needs of infant boys, teen-age girls, and adult men are quite different. The value of the goals is in identifying problems associated with food intake, which have become public health hazards.

Low Levels of Teen-Age Nutrition

Surveys indicate that teen-age girls consume the least nutritious foods of any age or sex group. Old enough to choose their food, they choose candy bars far too often.

Teen-agers eat too much sugar. Sugar contributes to tooth decay and obesity—and most Americans consume about 128 pounds of sugar a year. How to we manage to eat so much?

To repeat, commercial food suppliers have developed the philosophy, "If a little bit is good, a lot is better." Look at any label and you'll see what I mean. Whether it's

sucrose (cane sugar)
fructose (fruit sugar)
dextrose
lactose (milk sugar)
brown sugar
honey, or
corn syrup

it spells sugar. Sugar is too available, too cheap, and too good. And most of the time we don't even know when we're eating it.

In a 1978 issue of a popular consumer magazine, comparisons were made of items with reference to their sugar content. Surprisingly, certain seemingly non-sugared foods were found to contain a higher percentage of sugar than foods that were primarily thought of as sweets. For instance, Russian dressing could contain more sugar than a soft drink, non-dairy creamer more sugar than a chocolate bar, and ketchup more sugar than chocolate ice cream.

Sugar has four calories per gram. You can ingest your daily caloric requirements very easily without approaching your nutritional needs when you eat a lot of sweets. A piece of chocolate cake ranges anywhere from 400 to 500 calories. That is approximately one fourth of the normal daily caloric requirement for most teen-agers, and if you're dieting, it is at least one third. Meanwhile, it has supplied very little nutrition. Presweetened cereals contain the same exact amount of nutrients as unsweetened cereal, but 50 percent more calories.

In my practice, I see several problems with sugar. If you have a tendency to gain weight, you gain far more rapidly with sugar than with any other class of foods, including fats. This is because of the high concentration of calories and their palatability.

A lot of chronic fatigue in female teen-agers is related to their intake of refined sugar. Sugar is supposed to supply energy, but I believe that in excessive amounts it has the opposite effect. Too much sugar acts almost like a poison to the system of the overweight teen-ager. Once I withdraw the high-sugar foods from her diet, she not only feels better, but looks better and performs more efficiently—after the initial withdrawal jitters (like an addiction).

There are those who say that other types of sugars do not cause the same problems as table sugar. Since all sugars are ultimately broken down into glucose in the body (at a slower or faster rate), I don't see any metabolic difference. They differ only in caloric content, their degree of sweetness, and their taste.

Honey has been the biggest nutritional hoax perpetrated on the American public, and people who should know better have swallowed the myth (and the honey). I once saw a friend of mine, a brilliant internist, strolling in the local mall chewing on a piece of honey-dipped pineapple. When I reproached him, he defended honey as "nothing but fructose, which doesn't require insulin to metabolize it." The only advantage to fructose is that because it is sweeter, you use less of it.

Meanwhile, it is still *sugar*—from flowers instead of sugar cane—but sugar, nonetheless.

As for the nutrients that honey is supposed to supply, try eating 46 pounds of it for your daily requirement, or even 5 pounds for some of your vitamins. The nutritional composition of honey is minimal, and its use is only justified if you like the taste. (P.S., it's no more *natural* than sugar.)

Fast Food and Nutrition

Teen-agers eat too much fast food. How bad are fast foods? One top nutritionist says, "Humbug, so what if the kids eat McDonald's every night? Just add a salad and they have a balanced meal." Another argues, "There's nothing wrong with eating pizza—it's quite nutritious. After all, what is it? A piece of bread, some tomato sauce, and cheese. You have adequate amounts of protein, carbohydrate, fat, vitamins, and minerals."

That fast food is good food no longer seems arguable. In fact, my patients have children who eat more balanced meals at the local hamburger chain than they do at home. The problem isn't nutrition or cost—it's calories! One meal of a hamburger, French fries, and a shake can total 1,100 calories. That's a whole day's share of calories if you are on a diet. Only half a pizza with any meat topping will also finish you off for the day.

Let's look at some of the calorie counts for the popular fast-food chains.

Arby's

	Calories
Junior Roast Beef	240
Roast Beef	429
Turkey Sandwich with dressing	402
Super Roast Beef	705

Arthur Treacher's Fish & Chips

	Calories
Fish, Chips, Cole Slaw	
3-piece dinner	1,100
2-piece dinner	905

(Just think, if you have a cola with this meal, you would get 200 more calories. If you have a dessert, you're already off the diet chart!)

Baskin-Robbins

	Calories
1 scoop of ice cream with sugar cone:	
Chocolate Fudge	229
French Vanilla	217
Rocky Road	204
Butter Pecan	195
Chocolate Mint	189
Jamocha	182
Strawberry	168
Mango Sherbert	132

(Of course, it is easy to see from this list that chocolate always comes out on top calorie-wise. Too bad! Sherbet adds up to only about 30 calories more than some of the more caloric fruits such as bananas and apples, and will certainly not ruin a diet. It may, however, trigger a craving for more refined sugar.)

Burger Chef

	Calories
Hamburger	250
Double hamburger	325
Super Chef	530
Big Chef	535
French fries	240
Chocolate shake	310

Burger King

	Calories
Whopper	630
Whopper Junior	285
Double hamburger	325
Hamburger	252
Cheeseburger	305
Hot dog	291
Whaler	744
French fries	220
Chocolate shake	365

Colonel Sanders' Kentucky Fried Chicken

	Calories
15-piece bucket	3,300
1 drumstick	220
3-piece special (Includes chicken, mashed potatoes, gravy, cole slaw, roll)	660
2-piece original	595
3-piece original	830

Dairy Queen

	Calories
Small dipped cone	160
Large dipped cone	450
Small sundae	190
Large sundae	430
Hot Fudge Brownie Delight sundae	580
Banana split	580
Parfait	460
Dilly bar	240

Dunkin' Donuts

	Calories
Plain cake	240
Plain honey dip	260
Chocolate honey dip	250
Yeast-raised	255
Honey-dipped	275
Add for fillings	50

Hardee's

	Calories
Husky Deluxe	525
Husky Junior	475
Fish sandwich	275
Hot dog	265
French fries	155
Milk shake	320
Apple turnover	290

Howard Johnson's

	Calories
Small cone	186
Medium cone	247
Large cone	370
Sherbert	136
Fried clams (7 oz. package)	357

McDonald's

	Calories
Egg McMuffin	312
Hot cake, sausage, syrup	507
Hamburger	249
Double hamburger	350
Cheeseburger	309
Quarter Pounder	414
Quarter Pounder with Cheese	521
Big Mac	557
Fillet of Fish	406
French fries (small)	250
Hot apple pie	265
Chocolate shake	317

Pizza Hut

	Calories
Cheese pizza (thin crust)	1,030
½ of 13" pizza (thick crust)	900
½ of 15" pizza (thick crust)	1,200

White Castle

	Calories
Hamburger	164
Cheeseburger	198
French fries	219
Onion rings	341
Milk shake	213

How can the dieting teen-ager deal with fast-food restaurants?

If the whole family wants to go to a certain restaurant, and it's "there or nowhere," there are ways of coping. You don't have to break your diet or be depressed. You might be lucky and find one that has a salad bar.

If not, get the largest hamburger with mustard, ketchup, and no "special" sauce. Take off the top of the roll and use the bottom to push the hamburger in your mouth. You can have either a small order of French fries or a shake. REMEMBER, YOU CAN'T HAVE BOTH. Decide on the taste you want—sweet and cold or salty and crunchy.

If you pass an ice cream store on the way home, you can have frozen yogurt or a soft ice cream in a cup. If you are dieting, forget cones! If you really want a sweet, crunchy cone, just get one without ice cream. A 47-calorie sugar cone or a 24-calorie plain cone are diet bargains. I order empty sugar cones many times, and nobody even raises their eyebrows.

Keep three things in mind when eating fast food: (1) keep it plain—what you see is what you get; make sure there are no mysterious sauces on the meat (they're always worth a few hundred calories), and no fried coating on the fish (another few hundred calories); (2) if you know where you are going, take a cucumber or green pepper in your pocketbook to take the edge off your hunger; and (3) be grateful that most places now have diet soda.

Roller Coaster Eating—In Search of the Optimum Diet

Poor choices and frantic dieting give teen-age girls "roller coaster" eating habits.

A diet should be composed of a variety of foods to protect against the deficiency of any one substance and should meet the allowances recommended by the Food and Nutrition Board, National Academy of Sciences—National Research Council.

It is my feeling that during the teen years, a diet for weight loss and maintenance should be rich in *protein*. Protein is essential in diets for the following reasons:

1. It is necessary to body maintenance and growth.
2. It cannot be supplied by carbohydrates and fats, so it must be ingested.
3. There are no available protein stores in the body, so it has to be replenished constantly.

Like carbohydrate, protein supplies four calories per gram, but it is much more difficult to break down. In fact, it requires energy to break it down (called the specific dynamic action of protein), and in using this energy, it raises body heat or basal metabolic rate (BMR). Therefore, eating protein actually makes your body perform more efficiently.

Protein is made up of building blocks called amino acids. Twenty amino acids exist in nature, and the body can manufacture all but about eight from carbohydrates and nitrogen. These eight are called *essential amino acids* because (1) the body cannot manufacture them by itself, and (2) they are necessary for body maintenance and growth.

Animal products such as meat, eggs, cheese, and milk supply the essential amino acids and are called *complete proteins*. Vegetables, grains, and fruit, however, do not supply all the amino acids. Most plant proteins are combined with carbohydrates. That's why in a vegetarian diet the carbohydrate load must be high in order to get an adequate protein intake. The only pure protein found in nature is in egg whites. During the first 6 months of life, milk is the greatest source of protein.

Protein requirements are estimated at anywhere from .5 grams to 1.5 grams per kilogram of body weight. An adolescent girl weighing 110 pounds would need anywhere from 50 to 70 grams of protein per day.

American diets are made up of about 20 percent protein, which on a worldwide scale is quite high. There has been a great deal of discussion about lowering the amount of animal protein in the diet because it is always associated with fat.

When I talk about a high-protein diet, I refer to dairy and meat proteins, as opposed to vegetable proteins. I like this diet for teen-agers because:

1. It fills them up and sustains them for longer periods of time.
2. It makes them chew.
3. It gets them away from carbohydrates. Their appetites are not stimulated as much, and there is not as much of a tendency to overeat.
4. It is rare that someone will become fat on protein alone. You seem to be able to eat a lot more protein than carbohydrate without gaining weight.

No chapter on nutrition would be complete without mentioning fiber. This is an indigestible carbohydrate that adds bulk to bowel movements.

Fiber, or roughage as it used to be called, stimulates the bowels. Researchers have investigated certain groups of people whose diets were high in fiber and low in fat, and they found that there were fewer incidents of cancer of the intestine.

Many teen-agers don't get enough fiber because they prefer soft foods that require less effort to eat. I feel very strongly that fiber not only helps regulate bowel movements, but also helps eliminate certain intestinal or digestive problems related to irritable colon or spastic colon. Perhaps fiber will ultimately be a factor in reducing the risk of cancer of the bowel.

Here are some tips on how to keep your diet high in fiber:

1. Get some unprocessed bran in a health-food store and occasionally sprinkle it on a salad.
2. If you scramble two tablespoons of unprocessed bran into two eggs and fry them, they will puff up like a pancake, which you may eat with a little diet jelly. It tastes so fattening that you would never guess that it was a perfectly acceptable diet food.
3. Serve raw fruits unpeeled, and when you eat grapefruit, peel it like an orange so you get a lot of the membrane.
4. Use bran flakes as one of your choices for breakfast.
5. Sprinkle some bran on chicken when you are baking it.
6. Don't peel the strings off your celery.

Vitamins

The teen-ager who often shortchanges protein on a diet also shortchanges certain essential vitamins and minerals.

Fat-Soluble Vitamins (*Vitamins that Dissolve in Fat*): *The Look Better Vitamins*

Vitamin	U.S. RDA*	Function	Too Little	Too Much	Source
A	5000 international units	Helps you see both in dark and light; makes your skin great and teeth beautiful	Night blindness, skin infections, dry rough skin; slows growth	Joint pain, loss of hair, skin turns yellow	Green and yellow vegetables, yellow fruit, egg yolk, liver, cream, butter, whole milk, fortified margarine

*R.D.A.: Recommended Daily Allowance (National Research Council)

Vitamin	U.S. RDA	Function	Too Little	Too Much	Source
D	400 international units	Absorption of calcium and phosphorus, strong bones, *good* teeth and bones	Faulty bone growth (rickets)	Brittle bones	Fish, egg yolk, sunlight or ultraviolet light, yeast, fortified milk, butter substitutes
E	12 to 15 international units	Important to reproduction (in animals)	Anemia, breakdown of red blood cells	None known	Vegetable oils, milk, eggs, meats, fish, cereals, leafy vegetables
K	Unknown	Blood clotting	Tendency to bleed	Unknown	Green leafy vegetables, cheese, egg yolk, liver

Water-Soluble Vitamins (Vitamins that Dissolve in Water): The Feel Better Vitamins

Vitamin	U.S. RDA	Function	Too Little	Too Much	Source
B_1 (Thiamine)	0.5 mg per 1000 calories	Coenzyme in carbohydrate metabolism	Beriberi (disease of the nervous system), loss of appetite, digestive problems, heart problems, muscle pains, swelling	Rapid pulse, swelling	Pork, beef, liver, whole or enriched grains, beans
B_2 (Riboflavin)	0.6 mg per 1000 calories	Coenzyme in protein metabolism	Lip sores and cracks; burning, itching eyes	None known	Milk, liver, enriched cereals, cheese

Vitamin	*U.S. RDA*	*Function*	*Too Little*	*Too Much*	*Source*
Niacin	14–20 mg	Coenzyme in productive energy	Pellagra, weakness, scaly skin, mental disorders	(Began appearing with huge doses for mental illness). Flushing, heartburn, nausea, diarrhea, rapid pulse, fainting, high blood sugar, abnormal liver function, jaundice	Meat, peanuts, enriched grains
B_6 (Pyridoxine)	2 mg	Coenzyme in protein metabolism, good to prevent fluid retention	Anemia, hyperirritability, convulsions	Rare	Yeast, wheat, corn; liver, kidney, and other meats; limited amounts in milk, eggs, and vegetables
Folic Acid	400 mg	Coenzyme involved in formation of nucleoproteins, and hemoglobin	Anemia (reduced iron in blood cells)	Rare	Liver, kidney, fresh green leafy vegetables, asparagus
B_{12}	3 mg	Coenzyme in synthesis of protein, red blood cells	Special anemia, sore mouth and tongue, nervous, no period	No reports	Liver, kidney, lean meat, milk, eggs, cheese (not present to any measurable degree in plants)

Vitamin	U.S. RDA	Function	Too Little	Too Much	Source
C	45 mg	Connective tissue formation, strong blood vessel walls, necessary for wound healing, resistance to infection, and modification of the body's reaction to stress	Scurvy	Diarrhea, precipitation of kidney stones	Citrus fruits, tomatoes, cabbage, potatoes, strawberries, melon

Words you should know:

1. *Enzyme.* Organic substance capable of producing certain chemical changes in other substances without themselves being changed in the process. Their action is catalytic. Digestive enzymes act upon food substances to break them down. An enzyme is usually named according to the substance upon which it acts, with the common suffix, *-ase.*
2. *Coenzyme.* Enzyme activators.

I find the argument about whether or not to take a vitamin pill rather silly. Teen-agers who diet are always trying to cut out more food than they should. A vitamin pill seems the logical way to assure certain daily requirements.

Minerals

Minerals are inorganic elements widely distributed in nature. Their metabolic roles are as varied as the minerals themselves. Those found in your body may be grouped as "major minerals," which are present in large amounts, "trace minerals with a function," and "trace minerals without a function."

Major minerals include calcium, magnesium, sodium, potassium, phosphorus, sulfur, and chlorine. Calcium (Ca) is present in the largest amount, mostly in the bones. Calcium requirements for teen-agers are 0.8 to 1.2 grams per day. Dairy products supply most dietary calcium. One quart of milk contains 1,000 milligrams.

Phosphorus (P) is closely associated with calcium in human nutrition and bone-building, and both minerals occur in the same major food source, milk.

Potassium (K) is one mineral that is especially important in dieting. It is associated with fluid balance. It has a big effect on muscular activity, particularly the heart muscle. Often during the course of a diet a great deal of body water is lost, taking potassium with it. When blood potassium levels drop, weakness, light-headedness, and muscle irritability occur. (This also occurs with the use of diuretics or water pills.) Potassium-rich foods include oranges, bananas, spinach, white meat of chicken, and tomatoes. These should be included in a diet.

Sodium (Na) is also one of the more plentiful nutrients in the body. We are most familiar with it in salt (Na Cl), although almost everything has sodium in it. It has a great deal to do with body pH, cell membranes, and normal muscle tone.

Chlorine (Cl, sulfur (S), and magnesium (Mg) make up the other three major minerals.

The remaining minerals are called trace elements because they occur in the body in relatively small amounts and include iron (Fe), copper (Cu), iodine (I), manganese (Mn), cobalt (Co), and zinc (Zn).

6

The Best of Times and the Worst of Times

You've looked at yourself in the mirror, and it upsets you. The arguments in your house over your weight are straining your relationships with your family. Your brothers and sisters are making snide remarks about calling you a baby elephant. You can't get cute clothes at the discount houses anymore. There seems to be less material in the dresses. Salesladies direct you to larger sizes. You feet don't seem to move well on the tennis court; it feels like they're weighted down with lead. The guys don't call, or when you and a friend go somewhere, she comes home with the date that you want, and you get the date that no one wants. It seems you have no choice. You must lose some weight and see if that will improve matters.

There are some problems and some advantages to losing weight at this time in your life. You might say it's the "best of times and the worst of times."

Is This a Good Time (12 to 18 years old) to Start to Diet?

Yes	No
1. Hunger and desire to eat not as confused	1. Time of growth
2. "Forbidden-food syndrome" not firmly established	2. Motivation and discipline lacking
3. Can't be bothered to fix own food	3. Must rely on others for food

4. Suggestible and does well following instructions
5. Fluid retention not yet a problem

4. Lack of knowledge about nutrition
5. Peer-group pressure
6. Activity level unpredictable

First the Good News

Hunger and Desire to Eat Not as Confused

Normally, animals eat when something in the brain says, "I'm hungry," or whatever the equivalent animal phrase is. The same thing was true for primitive man before he invented the concept of "time." This urge occurred at any point in the day, depending on the fellow's activity level and the amount of stored energy. He was hungry, he ate, and he stopped eating.

With the development of civilization, particularly in prosperous nations, the emphasis has fallen on food for pleasure, rather than food for survival. We have become "food-suggestible," which means we frequently eat because we feel like it, not because we are hungry. Are you food-suggestible?

1. After a big meal, can you be persuaded to eat a dessert if it looks particularly good?
2. When you are sitting and watching TV, and they show some particularly delicious dish being prepared, do you find yourself walking to the refrigerator?
3. When you're walking down a busy street and you see a bakery, are you tempted to go in and buy something even though you were not hungry before you saw the bakery?

If you have a weight problem, you've probably answered "yes" to all three questions.

The overweight female is (no surprise) far more food-suggestible than the female of normal weight. She has a more heightened awareness of the taste, smell, and sight of food and can be persuaded to eat more even when absolutely full. Many times this behavior is so instinctive that she doesn't realize what she is doing.

After eating this way for a long time, she loses the ability to know when she is really hungry or merely aroused. I hope this hasn't happened to you. Most of the teens I have advised still eat because they are hungry, and this is, indeed, the proper cue. (See *Behavior Modification*, Chapter 7.)

What can we do to prevent this mixup of signals? Stop regular snacking between meals. One snack when you get home from school is sufficient to satisfy real hunger and to keep your blood sugar normal.

If you keep snacking, the snack periods get longer and longer until they run into mealtimes. Then you are not hungry at meals so you don't eat, and then you become hungry two hours later and start snacking. It becomes a cycle and wham!—you've gained 10 pounds, or at least you haven't lost an ounce.

Note the way many thin people eat. They might eat much more than some overweight people, but they eat at more appropriate times.

One clinic recently studied the relationship between actual time and eating. The participants were put in closed rooms and allowed to eat when they wanted to. Watches, clocks, and radios were removed from the research area so nobody had any idea what time it was. They could not even watch the sun.

It was fascinating to see that overweight people had absolutely no internal time clocks. They missed lunch by an hour or so because they didn't think it was lunchtime. By contrast, the others seemed to be extremely well-regulated, eating at proper times because they could distinguish between a real and false sense of hunger.

Therefore, an excellent way to regulate your hunger is to take your meals by the clock. If your schedule is so haphazard that you can't eat at the same time every day, then at least keep a precise interval of time between meals—say, five or six hours. You should be able to eat three good, satisfying meals, but you must *eliminate* between-meal nibbling or limit it to the lowest-calorie foods (fresh vegetables or, occasionally, one piece of fresh fruit). This way you can be pretty sure which signals are real hunger and which merely the urge to eat.

"Forbidden-Food" Syndrome Not Firmly Established

If a girl has overweight tendencies, from the time she understands what food is until the time she is an adult, she will associate certain foods with the words *bad, naughty, no-no*. As a result, these words become almost magical: *cake, pie, ice cream sundaes, gravies, sauces*—all are high in carbohydrates or sugars and starches. "Here you go, mmmm..." says a friend or relative to a heavy child, ladling chocolate sauce over a dollop of ice cream, "...but don't eat too much! It's *fattening.*" This scene is repeated until you can't help feeling there's something very precious about stuff you can eat only sometimes and just a little bit at a time. If we could have all the diamonds we wanted, they wouldn't be so expensive, and it's the same with fattening foods.

When you can get a lot of these foods (in a bakery or ice cream parlor) or when someone at home isn't looking, you may go "bananas" and eat as much as you can as fast as you can. This is called a "binge," and one of the reasons they're so frequent is the joyful, naughty emotion attached to forbidden foods from an early age.

How can you escape it? Clearly, the earlier you can convince yourself there's nothing special or "naughty" about chocolate cake, the better. You should learn to prize certain foods not because of their "naughtiness," but for other reasons: fruit because it's ripe and delicious (think of the crunchiness and juiciness of an apple); lettuce because it's thin and crisp; beets because they're tender and flavorful, and so on. To the overweight person, these qualities should be more attractive than sugar and starch content.

The earlier parents shatter the "mystique" of fattening foods, the less likely a fat teen-ager will "pig out" on packaged cookies.

While the "forbidden foods" theory is indisputable, it is overused. Many psychiatrists believe that people become overweight not because they're born that way, but because they eat "forbidden" foods to "get back" at their parents, friends, and the world. It's a form of defiance in which fat people punish themselves because they have a lot of anger and are afraid to communicate it directly to someone else. While this may be true in different degrees of some fat people, the urge to eat cake and keep eating it comes from other things.

I believe that overweight people can't tolerate carbohydrates for *chemical* reasons. A piece of cake, for example, will trigger something in their bloodstreams that produces a wild craving for *more* carbohydrates, until the urge to eat more and more cake becomes intolerable. Thin women and men don't have this problem because their body chemistries are different.

While overweight people may indeed be attracted to these foods because of their "naughtiness," that's usually not why they eat too much. You don't get fat by eating only one piece of cake; if you're afraid you will binge, convince yourself that you don't really want these foods.

Can't Be Bothered to Fix Own Food

Here's a jolly little plus: most teen-agers rarely feel like getting up from the table and making their own dinners, even if they don't particularly like what's being served. "Blech, vegetables," you may say, but you'll eat and fill up on them provided they're not too "gross." If your parents like balanced, low-fat meals, relax and enjoy not being tempted. If they don't, this can work against you.

Suggestible and Does Well Following Instructions

If I can get to you at an early enough age, I can do a good job convincing you how important it is to eat the right foods. That's why it's so crucial to develop sensible eating habits now. By the time you're older you'll be too suspicious if someone tries to take away certain foods and too used to eating the wrong things to change without difficulty. It's easier at this time for teens to follow positive suggestions, and that's all dieting is—a reinforcement of positive suggestions.

Unfortunately, young people can also be brainwashed in a negative fashion. I once met a girl whose family had totally convinced her that not using salt was the only way to diet. Nothing I said could change her mind.

The trick is for me to get to you first with the truth, when it's much easier to learn. My teen-age patients have more success losing weight than my adult patients, partly because they follow my instructions with more energy and determination once I have gained their trust.

Fluid Retention Not Yet a Problem

"Fluid retention" has both a medical and popular meaning. In this book I will refer to the popular meaning: the normal tendency of the female body to hold water rather than get rid of it. Some of the symptoms are a "bloated" feeling, pain and sensitivity in the breasts, and a swelling of the fingers and the abdomen. It is usually worse just before you have your period. It is caused by an increase in the female hormone *estrogen*.

You have young bodies, and your estrogen levels are uneven; this combination does not encourage fluid retention. However, you will have to deal with this problem soon, so I will discuss it briefly.

When a female diets, she expects to lose a certain number of pounds per week. If she sticks to the diet with real determination and doesn't cut back on exercising, she looks forward to that reward—say, a 2-pound loss. But there are weeks when the loss in weight will be offset by fluid retention. These are called "plateaus"—women don't lose an ounce, and sometimes they even gain slightly.

With periods the estrogen levels drop, the extra water leaves the body, and there is a significant weight loss. It is important to know about fluid retention because a woman may become upset when the scale doesn't reflect her efforts, and sometimes that's enough to make her stop dieting.

You must learn to expect "plateaus" eventually. They are perfectly normal and don't mean your diet isn't working.

Now the Bad News

It's a Time for Growth

This is only a disadvantage because some physicians and parents believe that early adolescents (10 to 14 years old) should never restrict their calories to the point of *losing* weight, but to the point of *maintaining* it. I don't agree. First, this is far more important for boys—who do most of their growing after 13—than girls, who have almost matured by that age. Second, most extra calories teen-agers eat are "empty" calories anyway—fattening junk food with no real nutritional value. They don't eat a lot of healthy food and their diets aren't well-balanced.

Safe weight loss can be attempted in early teens using a high-protein, low-carbohydrate, balanced diet in which all the calcium and vitamin needs are met for growth.

Motivation Lacking

Many teen-agers feel they have absolutely no reason to stop eating. They are comfortable within the family circle, and the whole world is an extension of that circle; everybody loves them, fat or not. As long as they have affectionate relatives, supportive friends, and can get into A-line dresses, they have no motivation to lose weight. It's too pleasant to eat. The first time many of my patients realized they were fat was after a routine checkup, when their school nurse told them they weighed too much. Often they were surprised.

Today many parents don't like to push their children. The only way most girls learn self-discipline is by developing talents like skating, piano playing, or dancing. These girls frequently have more success losing weight because their self-discipline can be extended to dieting.

Motivation may be greater in boys because physical skills are still more important. (Fortunately, this is changing. See Chapter 17.) Young girls want beautiful bodies, but they often don't want to work for them. They want to wake up in the morning and find beauty. That is wishful thinking. Boys seem to understand much better that you must work to get in shape for, say, wrestling or football.

Their greater self-discipline, plus the natural ability to burn calories more efficiently, make boys much more successful dieters. You'll often hear a girl say, "Gee, my brother lost weight so easily. He had to lose 15 pounds for wrestling, so he starved himself and the weight literally *fell* off him."

Must Rely on Others for Food

Have you seen this somewhere before? Check the plus column. Its the flip side of "Too Lazy to Fix Own Food," and it is a minus only if you have an uncooperative parent or relative. If you have a mother who puts spaghetti, macaroni and cheese, and creamed chicken under your nose every night, you often don't stand a chance of losing a significant amount of weight until you get away from that situation. My very first diet patient was a young girl with this problem. Her family lived on a farm where they were big eaters, and she just didn't want—or wasn't able—to refuse her mother's mammoth meals. Her successful weight loss came at the age of 21, and only after she had left home.

A Lack of Knowledge About Nutrition

Most schools teach four basic food types. They also talk about proteins, carbohydrates, and fats. They discuss calories, energy, heat, and work. They don't seem to know the difference between weight *loss* and weight *maintenance*, nutrition and diet, rapid weight loss and slow weight loss, and high-protein and high-carbohydrate diets. They don't often talk about what makes people fat or thin, and they never talk about why girls have a more difficult time losing weight. They don't even seem to realize it. They teach overweight in a unisex way.

But the schools aren't alone in their lack of understanding. Even in our country's most powerful institution, the military, there has been no allowance for the smaller number of calories females require for weight maintenance, let alone weight loss. The Armed Forces Diet, one of the largest standardized diet programs in the country, is over 4,000 calories and is obviously designed for men. Female recruits are expected to follow a diet that can cause enormous weight gain if they eat all their meals in a cafeteria or if their activity levels drop.

Restaurants are almost as bad. One of my pet peeves is the advertised "diet plate," which features cottage cheese, hamburger, rye crisp, and gelatin, or fruit salad, cottage cheese, and a little date-and-nut-bread sandwich This is not a diet plate. By themselves some of these things would constitute a diet plate; together they have too many calories. Diet plates average more than 500 calories; if you eat one for lunch and have a 300-calorie breakfast and an 800-calorie dinner, you're at the level of weight maintenance, not loss.

Peer Group Pressure

If your peers feel comfortable with you, they usually want to keep you from changing. They worry about what's going to happen if a fat friend suddenly becomes thin. Will she get stuck-up? Will she get too popular with boys? Sometimes your improved appearance threatens the way they see themselves.

They pressure you in other ways. If they go out and eat pizza, they want you to go our and eat pizza. If they go out for ice cream sundaes, they want you to go out for ice cream sundaes. Who can resist this kind of temptation? You have no reason to diet with friends who love you the way you are.

However, if you have friends who understand the way you feel about being overweight then peer pressure can become a positive force. Friends who encourage your dieting or even diet with you can give you the warm feeling that you are not alone. Of course, it can be very annoying when a super-thin girl friend decides to diet with you—that's just her way of calling attention to the difference between your weights.

Activity Levels Unpredictable

If my female patients ate normally and ran two to three miles a day, they would probably keep their weight within normal limits. If they dieted sensibly and jogged daily, they would lose weight. But getting a normal teen-age female to move is difficult; with an overweight teen-age female it is almost impossible.

These girls are always fatigued and tired, and somebody once suggested hopefully that they use all their energy in growing. But, to repeat, females complete most of their growth by the time they are 14 years old.

There are many reasons for female fatigue. One of them is basic: the overweight has naturally-low energy levels. (She will retain this "laziness" even after losing weight.) In addition, females are very sensitive to fluctuations in blood sugar and blood potassium levels, which are affected by dieting. They are also sensitive to premenstrual fluid retention and carbohydrate intake.

Females regard exercise as a chore, and just the thought of it often tires them out. When girls walk to school, they act like they've run a marathon. If their classes are far apart, they can come home exhausted. True, many teen-agers hold tiring jobs—waiting on tables, working in supermarkets—but that doesn't count in weight loss. Being tired is part of everyday living; only consistent exercise burns calories.

7

Choosing the Way You Want to Lose Weight

All right, you've decided that it's the best of times to lose weight. You must now find a plan that is right for you. Teen-agers are different; there is no "one diet that fits all," like a pair of panty hose. Any number of diets or *non*-diets can prove satisfactory, depending on your mood, the time of day, or whatever.

The most important thing is that when you choose a program for weight loss, you give it a fair trial, at least two weeks. Don't "diet hop!"

Although I'll save my real diets for later, here are some overall guides to the kind of dieting options available to you. Find the one that best suits your own needs and lifestyle.

Informal Plans

Some teens don't like the idea of going on a fixed, rigid schedule of food intake. They prefer casual, more flexible plans for weight loss.

Cutting Out Junk Food. This is the most common informal diet. The problem is, how do you define junk food? Why should salted peanuts in a bag be classified as junk and cashews from a health-food store be called nutritious? Why should candied corn be junk and granola cereal (filled with sugar) be healthy? Why should pretzels be junk and a slice of bread necessary starch? Is everything packaged in cellophane bags junk food? Then are dried beef and raisins junk food? Are store-bought oatmeal cookies junk and homemade ones okay?

Even though the government has been kind enough to define junk food, junk-foodless diets are all different. Therefore, the results are not always predictable. Some girls will lose weight and others will not.

Another problem is that substituting good food for junk food does not always result in weight loss. Two apples substituted for a small bag of corn chips gives you the same number of calories.

Cutting Down. This is a popular informal diet also. If your family serves a high-calorie meal, you can cut down by mentally dividing your food portions into three parts and eating only two parts. Highly-motivated people divide everything in half and do the same thing. This method is only effective if you take a normal portion of food.

Remember, you only have to do this when faced with high-calorie food; salads and plain vegetables can be eaten freely.

Cutting down is another unpredictable way to lose weight, but it is a useful technique. When you are forced into a situation where you feel you must eat or when you don't want anyone to know you are dieting, then use the "rule of the third."

Eating Magical Combinations. There is a firm, unfounded belief that certain foods alone or in combination dissolve fat. I guess this is the eternal dream. Nothing causes a breakdown of fat except using it as energy, and that means not supplying energy through your mouth.

Grapefruit is the most common food that people have invested with magical properties. It was featured in one of the first crash diets published, obviously because it's good, filling, and low in calories. Until that time, it had not achieved the popularity of its sweeter sister, the orange, and I wouldn't be surprised if some clever public relations man from the grapefruit industry dreamed up the whole grapefruit diet.

Lecithin and kelp became very popular a few years ago when it was discovered that they contained B vitamins that were somehow related to the breakdown of carbohydrates. Hot water with lemon before meals has gotten a reputation for melting fat. There is also a myth that pickles are so low in calories that you actually lose weight by eating them. Forget fat-burning foods. They are fun to think about, but so far none have been discovered.

Eating the Same Food. Some kids feel they will lose weight by eating the same food at every meal. On some diets, for example, all you can have is skim milk and bananas, or steak, eggs, and tomatoes.

Actually, this method of losing weight is only valuable because it becomes so boring that you end up eating very little.

There can be physical problems connected with eating too much of one food. As I'll explain in the section on "food allergies," eating or drinking too much of one food often leads to a reaction which you wouldn't get if you ate only smaller amounts of that food. Too much lettuce might give you diarrhea; too many oranges, mouth ulcers; too many strawberries, hives; too much cheese, constipation; and so on.

You can purchase any number of liquid and solid meal substitutes, which lend themselves to a monotonous weight-loss plan. They may be substituted for one, two, or three meals a day.

One of my first successful diets involved the use of the only liquid supplement on the market at the time. I drank it for three meals a day for two weeks. When I finished, I had lost 10 pounds, but suffered from terrible gas pains. I later found out I was allergic to the milk that formed the base of the supplement. I never knew I had a milk allergy until I drank one quart per day for two weeks.

Sometimes the supplements taste so good that people eat them *in addition* to their meals and gain weight. I have a chocolate-covered, peanut-butter-flavored bar in my office that is sensational (as far as diet bars go). It has 280 calories and contains a good balance of nutrients. The last person I put on "the bar" diet actually developed a craving for them.

Eating the same food obviously has limited usefulness in long-term dieting, but might be an interesting device to get you started on a more important diet.

Three-Meal-a-Day Diet. Another common diet plan is eating three meals a day with nothing in between. Except. of course, weight loss depends on *what* you eat at each meal. For instance, if you have pancakes with syrup, sausage, and fried potatoes for breakfast; hamburgers, French fries, and a milk shake for lunch; and spaghetti, garlic bread, salad, and cake for supper, with nothing in between, chances are you won't lose weight. Aside from that, confining your eating to three meals a day is probably the best and most effective way to diet informally.

Formal Plans

If you are really serious about losing weight, it is important for you to go on a formal diet. Your diet should have a beginning and an end. You should get weighed at regular intervals and have some idea of the length of time you will be dieting.

Since most non-crash diets for teens lead to a loss of 5 to 8 pounds the first two weeks and then 1 to 2 pounds a week after that, you should be able to determine the approximate time you will be spending on a specific diet.

Starving: This is the most popular formal method of weight loss for teen-age girls. (I call it formal because it calls for a rigid plan of eating nothing.) It fits beautifully into their all-or-nothing, black-or-white philosophy, and even has "mystical" overtones. Some people think that you purify yourself by starving and that toxic chemicals flow out of your body and mind.

Starvation has its good qualities: it's cheap, it's easy, it's fast, and after a few days, you are not hungry. But think about the bad qualities: it's dangerous, it's boring, it's anti-social (unless someone is starving with you), and once you break it, you tend to overeat.

Starvation doesn't purify you; it makes you lose body water so that you urinate all day long. If that's purifying, you are purified every morning when you get up. The kidneys remove waste from the body, but passing more water does not necessarily mean removing more waste. In fact, when you lose vital minerals like potassium and sodium, which are necessary for muscle strength and if your level of these minerals drops too low, you feel washed out, weak, and shaky.

The worst thing about starvation is not the loss of water, but the loss of muscle. When the body is supplied with *no* calories, it begins to look for its favorite food—carbohydrate. There are only about 13 hours of reserve carbohydrate stored in the body. Once this is used up, the body must start to break down fat for energy. But fat is an emergency fuel and the body uses sugar in the muscle to protect its fat stores.

Long-term starvation (over a period of several months) can account for up to a 30 percent loss of body muscle. If you were to lose that much muscle in a short period of time, you would die. Of course, you lose this muscle gradually over a longer period of time, and the body compensates for the loss. But it's extremely unhealthy. You also deprive yourself of protein, which is necessary for rebuilding and repair. *You* are particularly susceptible to muscle loss because you are in a growing phase, and it is vital that you preserve maturing muscle quality.

A fast is boring and anti-social. Think of how badly you feel when you go out to eat with friends and can eat only a salad. Think of how much worse it would be to sit there with only a glass of water. You might think it's hard to limit yourself to turkey, vegetables, baked potatoes, and fruit for Thanksgiving, but what about just having a bottle of diet soda?

You won't be able to study. Why? You will think of food all the time—not even sweets, just food. When you wake up from sleeping you will remember dreaming of food. You will break the fast like a ravenous bear and probably regain very quickly all the weight you lost. I once saw a girl gain back 16 pounds in four days.

Some people call a juice diet a starvation diet, but it is not. Fruit juices are loaded with calories—a day's supply of orange juice can provide you with over 600 calories. That is not starvation. That is a high-carbohydrate, liquid diet, but you still don't get any protein.

I don't think you will do any permanent damage by fasting for a few days, but you'll feel lousy. A short period of starvation breaks up binge eating and brings your appetite back to normal levels very quickly. It also makes you feel thinner immediately because your stomach gets flat from the rapid water loss. However, these benefits can be achieved with other methods of dieting. Therefore, it is *never* necessary to choose a starvation diet.

Counting Calories. Most of the diets you read, like the one in this book or popular crash diets like Scarsdale, Mayo Clinic, and Ski Team, have reduced calories. You can devise your own calorie diet if you follow some of these rules.

You need 15 calories per pound per day to maintain your body weight. If you weigh 140 pounds, that means you need 2,100 calories per day. If you decrease that by 500 calories per day, you should lose about one pound a week. If you decrease it by 1,000 calories a day, you should lose about two pounds a week (this is not always absolute). Therefore, your average weight-loss level is 1,100 calories per day. In those 1,100 daily calories, you should try to include 55 to 70 grams of protein, one pint of skim milk (for calcium), two pieces of fruit, and an adequate supply of green, leafy vegetables. You should include two to three starch products (bread or cereal).

Suppose you eat 1,100 calories a day, but you are not losing weight? (This happens quite often.) Make certain that you are balancing your feedings. If you are, cut your daily intake by 100 calories for one week (have one less fruit or starch). Make sure your bread or starch is eaten in the morning—for breakfast or lunch—and not for supper. Eventually, you should be able to lose weight, even if you have to go down to 850 calories a day. Do not go below that level for any sustained period.

If you are still not losing, you may be eating too many carbohydrates (see next section) or exercising too little. Don't despair. Overweight people burn calories at different rates; if standard calorie diets don't work for you, you must define your own level of calorie expenditure by trial and error.

Calorie-counting is routine and boring, but gives predictable weight loss when you find the correct level.

Counting Carbohydrates. This has been a very popular method of formal dieting in the last fifteen years. Low-carbohydrate diets restrict carbohydrate intake to under 60 grams per day (the daily recommended carbohydrate level is 100 grams). In this way you are supposed to lose weight without counting calories.

To refresh your memory, high carbohydrate foods include cakes, pies, candies, breads, noodles, rice, and potatoes. Fruit is moderately high in carbohydrate, particularly grapes, cherries, and bananas. Low-carbohydrate foods are meat, eggs, fish, cheese, and green raw vegetables (except peas).

The classic low- or no-carbohydrate diet states that calories don't count as long as you don't eat sugar and starches. While that may not be entirely true, some very interesting things happen on this type of diet:

1. You are not as hungry.
2. There is little or no muscle loss so the largest proportion of your weight loss is body fat.
3. Many people claim they have more pep.

You might say, "Hey, that's the diet for me." But it doesn't always work. I have found it to be a great diet for teen-age boys and *very active* young females. However, telling most overweight girls that they can eat all they want of anything, even if it is protein, allows them to eat up to the level of calories where they don't lose weight.

Interestingly enough, if you keep carbohydrate levels suppressed, you usually don't *gain* weight; therefore, this type of diet is excellent for weight maintenance.

A few difficulties encountered on the high-protein diets include mild nausea, diarrhea, bad breath, headaches, and occasional weakness. However, these side effects can be alleviated by the addition of more carbohydrate to the diet along with two ounces of orange juice.

Why does a diet like this work when it obviously goes against all laws of thermodynamics? It works for a number of reasons. First, high-protein, low-carbohydrate diets depress your appetite, so even though you can eat all you want, you don't want all you can eat.

Second, it is felt by some people that when you follow a high-protein, low-carbohydrate diet (the two must go together), you create a large amount of partially burned fatty acids called *ketones* in the bloodstream. These ketones have no available carbohydrates to unite with to complete the burning cycle. Because they are acids, they upset the delicate acid-base balance of the body. Since the kidneys must prevent the blood from becoming too acidic, they filter out the ketones so that you actually lose fat before it is converted into energy. (There are experts who violently disagree with this premise.)

Third, all foods have a specific dynamic action (SDA). That means that breaking them down (digesting them) raises body temperature. Carbohydrates have a low SDA because they are easily digested and metabolized for energy. Fat has higher SDA, but protein has the highest. Therefore, you burn more calories just by breaking down protein. Again, some experts claim that the difference in SDA is negligible.

Criticisms of high-protein, low-carbohydrate diets are that it is unbalanced, monotonous, and too high in fat (because it allows unlimited meat and eggs). Whatever experts claim, there is no question that you can eat a large amount of protein and not gain weight. That is the principle behind my High Calorie Weight Loss Diet, where I allow you to eat all the meat or fish you want at supper. I must admit that this has backfired when girls consume over a pound of meat nightly. They don't lose weight, but they don't gain either.

I recommend a combination of calorie *and* carbohydrate counting. The classic high-protein, low-carbohydrate diet includes meat, fish, eggs, cheese, green and yellow vegetables (except for corn and peas), grapefruit, and cantaloupe.

Protein Sparing Modified Fast Diet. (P.S.M.F.). This is the most radical and difficult of the formal weight reduction diets and should be attempted only in cases of gross obesity (in excess of 60 to 70 pounds) and only under the closest medical supervision. It resembles fasting in that it is an all-or-none diet.

But it is far better than starvation because Protein Sparing Modified Fasting means *starvation with the addition of protein*. I told you that starvation was bad for you because you lose too much body muscle and don't replace it. This diet supplies you with 60 to 70 grams of liquid or solid protein to replace your body protein, plus vitamins, calcium, and potassium.

In addition to 11 to 12 ounces of meat or fish daily (or a liquid protein), you may have water, diet soda, club soda, decaffeinated coffee, weak tea, and clam juice, plus vitamins and minerals.

It is not recommended for young teens (12 to 15), but I have seen it work effectively on 16- to 20-year-olds who weigh more than 200 pounds.

You must have, in addition to the diet, a very good program of medical supervision, supportive therapy, nutritional education, behavior modification, assertiveness training, and exercise.

This is obviously a diet for very few teen-agers; but for the grossly obese teen-ager who is unable to lose weight on any other diet, it is a fast, effective, and (in the right hands) safe way to lose weight.

The Three-Meal-a-Day Diet. Although I discussed this way of dieting as an informal method, I liked it so much, I formalized it. If you like the idea of three-meal-a-day dieting, see Chapter 11 and try the Carefree Diet.

Diet Groups. Diet groups represent formal diets. Most teen-agers I know like to diet alone or with a friend (team dieting); they don't enjoy "exposing themselves" to strangers. Also, their slow weight loss often puts them at a disadvantage when compared to adult dieters. Until now, diet groups have not been geared to teen-agers, but I think it's just a matter of time before the more commercial groups start teen-age chapters. The support of the peer group could be beneficial.

Sometimes mothers bring daughters to groups, but mothers and daughters make terrible dieting partners. Most of the time the mother loses weight faster, which often upsets the daughter enough to drive her off the diet.

Early in my practice, I made the mistake of running several groups for obese females in which there were no age limits. There was one quiet, shy 15-year-old girl, Diane, who blossomed in the group. Her weight loss was excellent, but even more important, she became a more confident person. One day, her mother, who was also a patient of mine, asked me if she could join the group. I told her that there might be some problems, but she insisted it would help her. I reluctantly agreed to let her participate, but only if Diane didn't mind. "Diane and I have a wonderful relationship," she said, "We do everything together." So the mother joined the group.

What happened next I entitle, "The Downfall of Diane." With each group session the mother attended, Diane became more and more withdrawn, while her mother became more enthusiastic and verbal. Diane's weight started going up as her mother's weight came down. This happened because Diane's weight loss was something she was doing by herself. For the first time, she was an individual. When her mother entered the group and took command, Diane slipped back into the role of the "child," and the "child" had always been overweight.

Behavior Modification

This is the most important and most significant of the non-diet approaches to weight loss. The original behavior modification clinics did not even include a diet.

Behavior modification came as an answer to traditional diet methods, which, as we all know, are unpredictable at best. Everyone was looking for some new magic. A psychiatrist from the University of Pennsylvania wrote an article on a method for treating obesity and called it *Behavior Modification*. It had been used in other areas of habit control, but never in weight control. When I read the glowing report, I rushed to the first behavior modification course I could find, hoping to discover the answer to overweight in this exciting new discipline.

What I found was a lot of artificial language around concepts as old as dieting itself. What I also found was another way for physicians to get rid of the responsibility for treating overweight (which they generally don't like to do) by handing it over to any paraprofessional who would take it. Behavior modification is not the answer for overweight, but it is somewhat successful as an adjunct therapy in weight loss and is particularly valuable in weight maintenance.

In essence, behavior modification talks about *cues*, which are triggers that make you act in certain ways; behavior, which is the action you take as a result of the cues; and outcome. In normal people

cue = hunger
behavior = eating
outcome = satisfaction of hunger and no weight gain

In overweight people, the cue could be *hunger*, and also *tension, boredom*, or *anxiety*. Behavior could be *eating normally*, but usually overeating or *eating high-calorie food*. Outcome could be *satisfaction of hunger*, but also *continuation of hunger and weight gain*.

One way to handle this is to modify or change the behavior so that the outcome is changed. Another way to handle it is to analyze the cues that are leading to the behavior and make them lead to activities other than eating.

Since all the studies indicate behavior modification's greatest success rate has been with teen-agers, I have liberally sprinkled this book with all kinds of behavior modification suggestions.

Special Considerations

Taking Diet Pills

There are four kinds of pills commonly associated with dieting: diet pills to curb appetite, both prescription and non-prescription; diuretic or water pills; and thyroid pills. There are also over-the-counter diet aids. No book on dieting would be complete without mentioning all.

Over-the-counter diet aids. These need no prescription and include diet candies or wafers that can be taken with a glass of water when you are hungry. They are supposed to satisfy your desire for sweets, give you energy, and fill you up. In many cases they do exactly what they are supposed to do, at least temporarily. Sometimes, however, they taste too good, and girls eat them like candy. Then they eat most of their food, too, and lose no weight.

Non-prescription diet pills. These are usually very small doses of the antihistamine decongestant *phenylpropanolamine*. They have been declared safe by the FDA and are useful in curbing appetite. They are sometimes combined with caffeine, to give you pep, and a local anesthetic, to dull the taste buds on your tongue.

They are so useful that some drug companies are selling them to doctors who do their own drug dispensing (a practice far too common with diet doctors). If you buy these pills from your drugstore, they come with a specific diet. If you wish, you can take them in conjunction with any diet in this book.

Prescription medication. If you want to send a roomful of doctors into orbit, just mention giving diet pills to teen-agers. Diet pills are usually amphetamines, or uppers. One of the strongest diet pills is sold for staggering prices on the illegal drug market under the name "Black Beauties."

When amphetamines were first on the market, they were used to overcome depression, not appetite. They were given to people who were so depressed that they couldn't move around or concentrate. Amphetamines made them peppy and alert, but after those effects wore off, the people would be more depressed than ever. It became obvious that they were the wrong pills for depression, but someone noticed that they also decreased appetite. So "diet pills" were born.

Amphetamines stimulate the central nervous system. They elevate blood pressure and cause overstimulation, restlessness, and headaches, but they do decrease appetite. However, the potential for abuse has become so strong that the federal government has stepped in to regulate them. There is now a warning on amphetamines which reads:

> Amphetamines have a high potential for abuse. They should thus be tried only in weight reduction programs for patients in whom alternative therapy has been ineffective. Administration of amphetamines for prolonged periods of time in obesity may lead to drug dependence, and must be avoided. Particular attention should be paid to the possibility of subjects obtaining amphetamines for non-therapeutic use..."*

There are a group of pills on the market called low-dose amphetamines, or nonamphetamines, that are quite effective in lowering appetite, but cause little or no stimulation. These can be useful in *short-term* (8 weeks) therapy for the treatment of weight reduction. The usefulness of any amphetamine must be weighed against possible risks inherent in the drug. The symptoms of "speeding" you get with an amphetamine—the "hyper" feeling—is not pleasant, and the subsequent "crash" can be devastating. Frankly, I can't see why anyone could possibly like the feeling.

*Physicians' Desk Reference.

Most teen-agers do not need diet pills; they are content to fill up on low-calorie food if it is available. They seem to be able to differentiate real hunger from craving much better than adults.

Diet pills may be off the market by the time this book is published. A group of legislators has been trying to ban them for a long time. It's too bad, because I feel they have a definite place in the treatment of obesity in well-selected, well-motivated patients who must bring their daily calorie requirement down to hardship levels (below 1,000 calories) for very long periods of time.

Diuretic or water pills. These are used to alleviate water retention. There is no question that weight loss comes to a grinding halt the week before your period and that it is due to estrogen-stimulated fluid retention. But this fluid retention is a far more significant problem in adults and is minimal in teens. Teen-age girls who feel bloated before their period need only to decrease salt and caffeine intake and take 150 mg of vitamin B_6 daily. Only if you suffer *severe* mood swings or irritability and depression should a diuretic be considered two or three days before your period.

Thyroid pills. The thyroid gland sits at the base of your neck and secretes thyroid hormone, which is necessary for the burning of energy. If your thyroid cannot secrete enough hormone, you feel cold and tired, suffer from dry skin, and have difficulty losing weight. Overweight girls have some of these symptoms, but most of their thyroid tests are normal.

There are a certain number of people who have all the symptoms of hypothyroidism (insufficient thyroid secretion), and yet their thyroid tests are normal. These people do well with small doses of a thyroid compound called Cytomel. By "do well," I mean that on a normal diet they lose weight in a normal way.

Let me tell you about Myra. She was a 19-year-old Rhodes scholar who ran 10 miles a day and ate 1,000 calories a day. She was afraid to eat less because of her strenuous schedule, but she couldn't lose an ounce of weight. She was a bright, healthy, articulate female, 5 feet 5 inches tall and weighed 155 pounds. Her blood tests were *normal.* She came equipped with an elaborate diet sheet listing her food intake. As far as I was concerned, her diet was well-balanced and her calories evenly distributed. She did not skip meals or eat in between. She had lost no weight over a period of three months. She did, however, complain of dry skin and coldness. I decided to try a small amount of

Cytomel on her for a minimum of four weeks and told her to pursue her diet as before. Her weight dropped to 139 pounds, and she felt wonderful. She completed her weight-loss program uneventfully and was gradually withdrawn from thyroid replacement. Her weight has kept at normal levels.

Remember, the rare candidate for this medication is the girl who has tried all conventional methods of dieting for a reasonable length of time and has not lost weight. It is not a magic way to lose weight, and it only works if you combine it with a diet.

Taking Vitamins

Vitamin pills are often given as part of a diet program. I approve of their use in the female teen-ager because she is always trying to eat less than she should and often doesn't select the food that will be most useful to her. A vitamin-iron combination is good because growing girls can become anemic as a result of heavy menstrual periods and inadequate iron intake. One problem is that iron tends to be constipating. If this happens to you, you will have to try getting your iron from foods that contain an abundant supply.

Injections

Injections of any sort have no place in the treatment of overweight teen-agers. Any medicine that is going to be given to teen-agers for diet can be given by mouth. The most common injection in dieting is Human Chorionic Gonadotrophin (H.C.G.), which is given daily and is accompanied by a 500-calorie diet. This is a hormone of pregnancy and is supposed to make all fat readily accessible for burning when you diet. After studying it for some period of time, doctors discovered that it was the 500-calorie diet that was effective, and not the H.C.G.

Bypass Surgery

One of the newest and most startling methods of dealing with extreme obesity is bypass surgery. The teen-ager with over 100 pounds to lose could consider this. The stomach is made smaller, less than one half its original size, by sewing shut the bottom part. You eat less, lose your desire for high-carbohydrate foods, are filled up more easily, and are content to diet because you are not hungry. In fact, if you eat more than a few ounces of food, you throw up. Pretty drastic? Well, it is! But as horrible as it sounds, it has proved to be safe.

I was horrified by the idea of this type of surgery when I first heard about it. But now, when I see a teen-ager who is more than 100 pounds overweight walk into my office, I realize the odds are against her losing all of her weight. She will lose some—20, 30, maybe even 40 pounds—but she will still be obese. Her task is almost mind-boggling, and she rarely completes it. In these situations, this type of surgery should be considered. It should only be performed by the most qualified surgeon, someone who not only understands the technique, but also the postoperative management of the patient.

8

Getting to Know You

You have chosen a diet. You are ready to start immediately. Hold off a minute. Let's find out something about *you*. Buy a nice fat notebook (in a few months that will be the only fat thing about you) and start to get acquainted with yourself.

Getting to Know Your Physical Background

What was your birth weight? It is interesting to speculate on whether you came into this world with too many fat cells or they developed later. Experts are still trying to determine at what point you get your extra fat cells—in the first two years of your life, the first six months, or in the last trimester (three months) of your mother's pregnancy.

Were you breast-fed or bottle-fed? Many of my patients have no idea how they were fed as infants, but an overwhelming proportion of their mothers tell me they were bottle-fed. That could have been because 12 to 20 years ago, breast-feeding was not as fashionable as it is now. Although there is not a wide caloric difference between breast milk and cow's milk (cow's milk has more protein and less carbohydrate), breast-fed babies are less likely to be overfed. The baby stops sucking when she isn't hungry, rather than the mother stopping when she thinks the baby is full.

How was your appetite as a child? Were you a good eater, always cleaning your plate, or a finicky eater? Did you have to be bribed with goodies to eat regular food?

Were you ever thin? When did you stop being thin? Many girls never had a weight problem until something happened that decreased their normal activity level. For example, you might have had your tonsils out. You came out of the hospital with a terribly sore throat and your family fed you ice cream to soothe your pain. You ate gallons of ice cream and lay in bed. By the time you were up and around, you had started on the road to being fat.

Getting to Know Your Family

How does your family handle your weight problem? Do they ignore it? Perhaps they are afraid of hurting your feelings. Nice people, but misguided.

Or do you think they ignore it because you look good to them no matter what shape you are in?

Or have they tried to discuss it with you, at which time you ignored them?

Maybe they are given to extremes of behavior. They may push food on you and say, "Eat! Eat! It's good" or "The whole world is starving, and you leave half your macaroni.'

They could be parents who constantly pick on you. "Stop eating!" "Don't eat that!" "Should you really be eating that?" "You're really too fat for that!" Most teen-agers rebel against this type of parent. Unfortunately, the most natural way to rebel against someone who always picks on you to diet is to eat.

Decide whether or not you can work with your parents, whether or not you trust them to help you lose weight. If you can't work with them, your diet could be more difficult.

Getting to Know Your Head

It is very important to understand yourself at any time of your life, and perhaps even more so when you are about to embark on a diet. The most important issue is *feelings*. How do you *feel* about being overweight?

Are you angry? If so, at whom is your anger directed? Are you angry with your mother for feeding you too much? Or your parents for giving you fat genes? Or your friends for being so thin and being able to eat everything they want? Or are you really just angry at yourself for not having the self-discipline to stick to a diet?

Anger is not a positive emotion; it takes a lot of energy and leaves you very tired. When dieting, you will need energy to exercise sound judgment. You do not have any extra to waste on being angry.

Are you indifferent? Do you wonder why everybody is making such a fuss about your weight? Perhaps you tell yourself you couldn't care less. I have seen very few teen-age girls who really couldn't care less. As a matter of fact, the most indifferent girls often feel the worst about their weight. It is much better to admit to yourself and others that you are having a problem than to pretend you don't care. In an age where the tiniest pimple on the chin can cause you tremendous humiliation, 10 to 20 pounds on the hips must do the same thing.

Investigate your indifference and see what it means. You might be surprised to find some very strong emotions that should not be hidden.

Are you embarrassed? Why? Are you afraid to be seen? Unfortunately, it's very hard to hide being overweight. You can get bad teeth capped, a big nose fixed, or thin hair teased, but when you are overweight, "it all hangs out." Therefore, you might as as well carry it off in the best possible fashion. Whether or not you want to lose weight, if you are fat, don't keep your head down and hunch up your shoulders. Walk tall and *wear clothes that fit.*

Are you depressed? Depression, like anger, is a tiring emotion. Unlike anger, it is something we can't control. True depression is manifested by difficulty going to sleep, early morning awakening, and would you believe ... loss of appetite?

Crying does not necessarily signify true depression. You are probably crying because you feel sorry for yourself. You feel resentful. You feel angry that *you* have to go through all this trouble to be thin. You are crying because you can't wake up one day and be beautiful and slim. You are crying because you have to exert constant self-discipline and nobody likes to do that, particularly in the area of food.

Are you ashamed of your weight? Don't be! It is not a sign of inadequacy or weakness. It is not a sign of stupidity. It does not mean that you're a pig.

Overweight indicates that you are unwilling or unable to accept the caloric restriction that nature has imposed on your body. Living with those restrictions is not an easy task. I have adult patients who are remarkably successful in all professions and have overcome many kinds of problems, and yet in the area of food, they are unable to succeed. They are, however, bright, articulate, and nice human beings. They don't have to be ashamed.

Try to understand yourself. Control some of the emotions that can be controlled. Work off anger and depression. Investigate the roots of indifference and overcome embarrassment and shame.

Getting to Know Your Diet History

When I see a new patient, I take a diet history. Psychiatry has a term called "Repetition Compulsion," which is when people repeat the same mistake over and over. Most dieters tend to repeat their mistakes. Perhaps if you take your own diet history, you will not repeat the same mistakes.

Outline the major diets you have gone on (not the little starts and stops), when you went on them, how long you stayed on them, and which were most effective and easiest (low carbohydrate, counting calories, and so on). Did you get weighed before you started and after you finished (most teen-agers do not; they just "feel thinner")? How many pounds did you lose? Why did you stop dieting?

This is important information. For instance, you might realize that you have never gone on a formal diet plan. You took an idea from here and an idea from there, and when you didn't get the kind of results you thought you should, you simply dropped the whole diet.

You might realize that you lost the most weight when you ate several small meals and the least when you ate one large meal.

You might realize that you can eat bread in limited quantities, but once you start eating sweets, it is all over.

You might realize that you are a total flop at calorie counting; you resent it, it makes you angry, and it makes you eat more. Obviously that is not the kind of diet for you.

You might realize you lose weight beautifully on fad diets or fast diets, but when you finish them, you don't understand how to keep your weight down.

You might realize that you have the staying power to diet one day, one week, or one month.

You might realize that you diet like you live, in a haphazard, undisciplined style. You have to realize that diets must be orderly.

Analyzing these patterns can help you learn about your personality and keep you from repeating the same mistakes.

Getting to Know Your Eating Habits

Behavior modification points out the value of analyzing your eating habits. It teaches the three "R's" of successful dieting

R ecord keeping
egimentation
easoning

In fact, when it comes to food intake, record keeping is one of behavior modification's most important contributions.

When I used to ask my patients what they ate, the answer was always a little vague: "I don't know." Seldom did anyone remember their wildest binges, even if those binges resulted in obvious weight gains. The most striking fact was that even though these people were dealing with frustrating weight problems, they deliberately ignored concentrating on the who, what, where, when, why, and how of eating. Keep a record that answers these questions:

Who Is Dieting. You are dieting. You, the overweight teen-ager, not your mother, your brother, your sister, or your friend. Don't concern yourself with how they feel. You do the planning and the decision making. Once you've made up your mind to diet, you must think about yourself first.

What Are You Doing? You are on a weight-reducing diet. That means that in some way you are committed to reducing your food intake for the sole purpose of losing weight and looking and feeling better. If you cheat, you only cheat yourself. Remember that!

What Are You Eating? What kinds of food are you eating? Analyze the content of your meals and snacks. Are they natural foods? Are they foods made with sugar and flour? Are your meals high in starch and low in protein? Change the *type* of food you eat and you might control your weight effectively.

Take a food history. List foods that you absolutely won't eat, foods that you really love, and foods that you can tolerate. Check the vegetable list in Chapter 11 and determine your variety quotient (VQ).

Happily, diet success does not have to be related to the variety of food you eat. I have seen girls diet successfully on nothing but tuna fish, lettuce, and apples. A variety of food becomes important when you say, "I can't stand eating the same thing."

What Do You Do When You Are Eating? Talking with the family is fine, but avoid reading, watching TV, or talking on the telephone. You lose track of what you are putting into your mouth.

What Mood Are You In When You Are Eating? Are you eating when you are bored, tired, upset, or frustrated?

When Are You Eating? When do you do most of your eating? Is it during those two deadly dull hours between getting home from school and supper, when there is nobody home except a chocolate cake? Or do you wait until nighttime while doing your homework? Or do you start your affair with the refrigerator at 2:00 A.M.? Or do you snack between classes?

Where Are You Eating? I once had a secretary who was obese, but I never saw her eat. She gave me a ride home from work one day, and I discovered food in every available space in the car. Cookies behind the visor, corn chips under the seat, and empty donut cartons in the back. She was the mobile equivalent of what we call "closet eater"; she was a "car eater." She would have helped her weight loss program by biking to work (nowhere to hide goodies there).

Where do you do most of your eating? Chances are that it's not in the kitchen or dining room. Could it be in your bedroom, in the den, or even in the bathroom? How can you stop this?

Pick one place to eat—the kitchen table. Resolve that whatever snacking or eating you do, you'll do it *sitting* at that spot.

Why Are You Dieting? Because you are overweight and want to get thin, and dieting is the only possible way to get thin.

Why Are You Overeating. Food is a part of everyday life and obviously it is impossible to avoid it altogether. But the dieter must avoid unusual temptation. The first place to avoid temptation is in the home.

1.   Ask your mother to buy no food that presents a particular problem to you. If you love potato chips, ask her to switch over to another snack that the rest of the family enjoys.
2.   Ask that any favorite food brought into the home be placed out of your sight.

3. Freeze anything you might grab. The rest of the family can wait for it to thaw out, but if you are on one of your eating binges, it will be unavailable for immediate consumption.
4. Try to avoid helping yourself to food. Ask the person who serves the food to serve you a fixed amount. Ask whoever cooks to prepare only enough servings for the people who are eating.
5. Never sit and watch other people eat, particularly if you are fond of the food they are eating. It will make you feel like a martyr. Ask if you can be excused from the table and rejoin the family at the end of the meal.

How Are You Eating? Are you eating fast, gulping? Are you tasting your food? Do you eat junk all alone, or do you dine on gourmet food in the company of others? Ninety percent of you will answer the former. Do you eat at regular or irregular times?

You'll probably discover that you are an undisciplined, high-carbohydrate eater who gulps food down before you can even taste it.

1. When you eat, taste your food and appreciate it; don't gulp. Chew at least 10 time per mouthful.
2. Don't take a large plate and fill it up. Take a small plate and fill it up.
3. Don't take seconds.
4. Put your fork down occasionally during a meal.
5. Get into the habit of not cleaning your plate.
6. Try chopsticks. They are inexpensive and will definitely slow you down. They are also fun to use, particularly in Chinese restaurants.
7. Relax at meals. Don't get into any arguments. Try to enjoy the people you are eating with; even the most boring dining companion can have something valuable to offer.

Keeping a diary that answers these questions is exceedingly important, even before you start a diet. It will identify eating *errors*, so you can try to correct them. Keep the diary for about a month before you start on a diet. If you start one immediately before your diet, you will be on good behavior and won't know what's wrong with your eating habits until you stop dieting, and then it's too late. As you lose weight, go over your diary constantly to remind yourself of your weak areas.

Getting to Know Your Present Eating Habits

Record your present eating habits in the form of a chart. The first column should be titled *Food Eaten*; the second, *Time*; the third, *Location*; the fourth, *Feeling*; the fifth, *Normal or Abnormal Reaction* (mad at myself, and such). Write at the end of each day or you will forget. This way any indiscretions will be readily observable, and if you don't lose weight the way you thought you would, the record will give you the clue to why.

Getting to Know Your Future Eating Habits

The first diary was "Eating: Past"; the second, "Eating: Present"; and now a diary of "Eating: Future." The most universal traits that I have observed in teen dieters is their inability to plan for tomorrow. They refuse to *anticipate* food problems. They believe something magical will happen that will protect them from overeating. Not so! Diets take planning. You have to be one step ahead, always. Ask yourself ...

1. What is going to get in the way of my diet tomorrow?
2. How can I change that?

Don't let tomorrow find you unprepared. Most of us have a very good idea of our schedules, whether they involve going to school or work, staying up late studying for an exam, going over to a friend's house, or going out on a date. Try to deal with tomorrow today and you will have a much better chance of staying on a diet. Of course, unexpected things happen, but at least you tried.

Perhaps your schedule for tomorrow will say, "A visit to Grandmother." Do you realize that your grandmother prepares fattening food, and she's going to insist you eat it? You don't want to hurt your grandmother's feelings (this is a very common attitude, although nobody ever died from having their feelings hurt). What do you do? You anticipate the battle and concoct a strategy.

Bring her a surprise—a beautiful fruit salad, tossed salad, or a simple fruit dessert—and say, "Gee, Grandma, you are always preparing dinners so I thought I would help you out." Then be sure you eat what you brought.

Try to understand why refusing food makes you feel uncomfortable. You don't always have to accept food just because somebody offers it to you.

You could pretend that you are allergic to fattening food—if you eat it, you will break out in giant fat cells. You can say without feeling guilty, "No, thank you. I'd love to eat that, but it doesn't agree with me," or "I'm allergic to it." Anybody who has a weight problem is allergic to sweet and rich foods, so technically, you wouldn't be lying.

I would rather you say, "No, I'm sorry, I have a weight problem and eating that would make it worse," but if that embarrasses you, lie. Isn't it foolish not to give somebody an honest answer or a simple "no, thank you"?

9

Diary of a Fat Teen-Ager

6:45 A.M.—Alarm going off. Too tired to move. Too sick to move. Must be all those chocolate-covered peanuts I ate last night. Why did I eat the whole can?

7:15 A.M.—Breakfast. I'm not hungry. Too tired and sick to eat. I think I'll skip breakfast and go on a diet. This is a good start.

10:00 A.M.—So tired. This math class will never end. I wish it were lunchtime so I could relax. Wish my stomach would stop growling—everybody keeps looking at me.

11:30 A.M.—This cafeteria is a zoo. If I want to diet, maybe I should skip lunch and just have a soda. No breakfast, no lunch, and I'm not even that hungry!

1:30 P.M.—I'm starving. Something smells good. Oh! Sheila has a bag of corn chips. Can I have one? Another? These are great. How much do you want for the rest of the bag?

2:30 P.M.—I'm beat. What a day. Gotta get more sleep. So hungry. I'll make myself a salad when I get home from school.

3:15 P.M.—I'm home! Where's the salad? Oh! I have to wash all that lettuce and peel all those vegetables? I'm too hungry to do all that. What's around that doesn't need washing? There's Mom's chocolate cake. I shouldn't, but just a small piece. This is terrific! I can't stop eating this. Oh, my gosh! I ate half of it. I'd better go up and take a nap before I eat the rest.

6:00 P.M.—Oh, that was a good sleep. I'm still tired though. Too full to eat dinner, but I have to sit at the table with the family. No thank you, nothing for me. Well, maybe a few French fries. These are good. I can't let all this food go to waste. Pass the fried chicken.

9:00 P.M.—This science homework is hard. I better have some of those oatmeal cookies for energy.

11:30 P.M.—Can't sleep. Must be that long nap I took. I'll watch the late-night talk shows.

12:45 A.M.—Yum ... that pizza in the commercial looks great. Too bad it takes so long to make. We have some spaghetti and meatballs in the refrigerator. I'll have a plate of that.

2:00 A.M.—So full. I feel sick. Better go to bed. How will I ever get up in less than five hours? (Yawn) Maybe I'll start a diet tomorrow ...

What's Wrong With the Fat Teen-ager?

6:45 A.M.—It is common to feel sick after late-night eating. This is called the "night eating syndrome" and is characterized by large late meals, restless sleep with dreams, and in the morning, fatigue, loss of appetite, and mild nausea. You break it by reversing your eating pattern. Substantial breakfasts and light evening meals.

7:15 A.M.—Skipping breakfast is a terrible way to start a diet. It accomplishes nothing. Breakfast starts efficient energy production and is the one meal that the body metabolizes correctly. I encourage you to eat breakfast. Skipping it will not make you lose weight faster.

10:00 A.M.—The body is slow in producing energy without breakfast. Many people misinterpret a growling stomach for hunger. Actually, stomach contractions can be brought on by the sight or smell of food, even if you are not hungry. If your stomach is well-trained (if you are on a regular eating schedule), it rarely contracts between meals. Blood sugar levels are low at this time of day, adding to fatigue. Difficulty concentrating makes keeping awake difficult.

11:30 A.M.—Most overweight teens avoid school lunch. Perhaps they don't want to be seen eating. Again the teen is fooling herself: giving up lunch is no way to start a diet. Her appetite is now depressed because she is in a mild starvation state (this is what happens in starvation diets).

1:30 P.M.—This happens to the very overweight person who tries to diet in this fashion. Sight and smell stimulate the appetite, and dieters usually grab empty calories: high-carbohydrate food that does not satisfy and, in fact, stimulates the appetite. And there go 300 calories. She could have eaten lunch.

2:30 P.M.—Her blood sugar is down because of a high-carbohydrate snack. This leads to early fatigue and hunger.

3:15 P.M.—Impulse eating leads to weight gain. She should have planned ahead and cleaned the salad the night before instead of watching TV. It's too bad her family isn't cooperating. At least they could have hidden the chocolate cake. *Chocolate is probably the number one diet-breaker for teen-agers.* If it's any comfort, you start to lose some of your taste for chocolate by the time you are 40. Notice also how one piece is never enough. A thousand calories for that snack.

6:00 P.M.—Look at that long nap! If she keeps eating sweets, she will always be fatigued, and if she thinks her fatigue is due to lack of energy (that is, lack of food), she will eat more sweets. And she will never get to sleep at a reasonable hour. Then she sits at the supper table with no intention of eating, but the sight and smell of the food stimulate her appetite. Again, she reaches not for the salad, but for the most fattening food. She eats the chicken "because it's there." In all, she eats 800 calories for dinner.

9:00 P.M.—She feels fatigued. Of course. Too much of the wrong food, too little exercise. But she makes a common mistake again. She thinks she needs energy, so she eats sugar. This is just what she doesn't need at 15 pounds overweight. Her fat could have supplied plenty of energy: 200 or more calories.

11:30 P.M.—No wonder she can't sleep. She slept all day and hasn't done any real work. She's taking a chance watching late-night TV. It's going to make her hungry.

12:45 A.M.—It made her hungry and she had nothing low-calorie prepared. She picked the starch food again, spaghetti and meatballs: 500 calories.

She has eaten 2,800 calories, of which 70 percent is carbohydrate, and most were eaten late in the day. This is a terrible way to lose weight because you overload your digestive system just when your basal metabolic rate is going down. Girls who skip meals and eat only supper don't lose weight efficiently. Tomorrow morning she'll wake up exhausted and repeat the cycle.

Now Let's Try Getting Up

I will guide our teen-ager through the following day:

6:45 A.M.—You feel sick and tired and can still taste the spaghetti. Get out of bed anyway. Take a cool shower and do 10 jumping jacks.

7:15 A.M.—Eat a *small* breafast: a poached egg, a slice of dry toast, and tea.

10:00 A.M.—Still tired, but that's to be expected. Do some exercises in place; make a circle with your toes; put some pressure on the tight muscles in the back of your neck; relax.

11:30 A.M.—*Eat Lunch.* Get a plain salad, cottage cheese, fresh fruit. No *refined* sugar.

1:30 P.M.—If still tired, practice relaxing muscles; try to keep blood pumping. Use break time to walk briskly around school.

2:30 P.M.—You are getting hungry. Visions of chocolate cake dance in your head. You are pooped. You feel you need energy.

3:15 P.M.—You're home from school. Pig out on skim milk, cheese, raw vegetables, fruit. You can eat nothing else. Don't go to sleep. Clean your drawers (3 calories per minute) or set the table for your mother. Try to study now. Open the window wide if you feel lazy. Drink diet soda.

6:00 P.M.—You are falling asleep on your feet, but you are starved. Eat a good supper, avoiding only bread and rich desserts. This is your last solid food tonight. Go out for a short jog at 7:00 P.M. It will help burn off your supper.

9:00 P.M.—You're exhausted and starved. You may have the following: diet soda (not cola), nonfat milk, clam juice, tomato juice. Your stomach is grumbling, Ignore it.

11:00 P.M.—You're so hungry that you can't sleep ... sleep ... zzzzzz. And you have broken the cycle.

10

Principles of Dieting (Like It or Not)

Don't let anyone tell you that dieting is easy. Dieting is sometimes depressing and usually difficult, but it is something that has to be done if you have a weight problem and want to be thin. When I realized that I wanted to be a doctor, I knew I would have to take courses like calculus and physics, which I hated; there was no other way to get into medical school. There is no other way for you to get thin besides dieting.

Whenever a teen-ager goes on a diet, she has a tendency to want to make her own rules. Sometimes her own rules seem very logical, given what she *thinks* she knows about her body. But calorie burning is extremely complex, and the right way to diet may not always seem logical. When a teen-age girl diets, she must keep three very important principles in mind:

1. Total calories should be decreased
2. Feedings should be balanced
3. 30 percent of total daily requirements should be protein (meat, fish, eggs, cheese, or nonfat milk)

Decrease Total Calories

Many teen-agers tell me they diet by giving up junk food and then become very upset when they don't lose weight. I call that "passive dieting." Males can diet passively—they merely give up a snack or dessert and the pounds drop off.

A female can't do that; she must *actively* diet. She must decrease her calories significantly, sometimes below what is considered a healthy level. Many times I have had to decrease calories for dieting adults to starvation levels, but I *won't* do that with teens. Luckily, most teen-agers can lose weight comfortably on 1,200 calories per day.

Balance Feedings

Most teen-agers dislike eating on a regular schedule. Often they skip meals altogether. Meals should not be skipped. YOU DON'T LOSE FASTER IF YOU SKIP MEALS. In fact, it might even slow down your weight loss.

Look at the diary of our fat teen-ager (see Chapter 9). She skips breakfast because she wants to diet and isn't hungry, and she gives up lunch because she wants to save time and calories. But when she starts eating, she can't stop. Of course our teen-ager is an extreme example, but the girl who skips breakfast and lunch and eats only supper is also in trouble.

If this is hard for you to understand, look at this study in which four groups of women were fed a different number of calories daily, divided in different ways.

	Breakfast	Lunch	Supper	Total
Group 1	250	250	500	1000
Group 2	0	250	500	750
Group 3	0	0	500	500
Group 4	0	0	1000	1000

Which group lost the most weight? Group 1 lost about 2 pounds a week. Group 2 lost slightly less than 2 pounds per week. Group 3 lost 2 pounds a week. Surprised? The biggest surprise is that Group 4 lost less than 1 pound a week.

Dieting must have a certain regularity. Eating once a day actually slows down weight loss. Eventually the women in Group 4 would not have lost any weight, even though their total calorie count was low enough. This is because the female body can burn only so many calories in a given time period before it begins to store food as fat. In adult females the "magic number" seems to be 500, based on a three-meal-a-day plan; therefore, under normal circumstances, if you eat more than 500 calories at any one meal, you will store the excess calories as fat.

You might ask, "What about the calories we burn when we don't eat anything?" As I said before, if you don't eat anything, you don't use energy efficiently and don't burn as many calories as you expect. You will always store more than you burn if you eat only one meal a day, unless that one meal is exceedingly low in calories (around 500). Then you will lose weight, but you will feel like you are starving. And normal girls can only starve themselves so long; at the end of the starvation period there is usually a binge that abolishes the weight loss.

One of the biggest arguments that I have with teen-age dieters is over breakfast. "If I'm not hungry, why should I eat?" they ask. On the surface that seems logical enough, but according to body rules, it doesn't work. There are regular times to replenish energy. One of the most natural is after the longest period of food abstinence, which is sleep. Sleep is the time when the metabolic processes are slowed and reserve energy stores are used. When we wake up we need energy to start our system, energy generated by food intake. Giving up breakfast deprives the body of this needed energy. It can even slow weight loss down. When you eat breakfast, you do the following things:

1. You keep your blood sugar at a level where you can think more clearly.
2. You avoid midmorning fatigue.
3. You burn energy more efficiently, especially if you eat lunch and dinner at regular intervals.

I've heard all the arguments for not eating breakfast. They include:

> I feel sick in the morning when I wake up.
> Breakfast makes me sick.
> Breakfast makes me late for school.
> Breakfast makes my face break out.
> Breakfast makes me feel tired.
> The only food I like for breakfast is fattening.
> If I eat breakfast, I am hungry all day long.

If you've convinced yourself of any of these things, eating breakfast can make you resent dieting. I know very few teen-agers who jump out of bed full of pep and energy. Usually they fight for the last minute of sleep and drag themselves out of the house barely awake. The idea of eating breakfast when you can't even speak is not very appealing. I sympathize, but I believe that breakfast helps you to lose weight more quickly and efficiently and makes good nutritional sense.

Will eating late at night get in the way of losing weight? This is a question I hear quite frequently. Actually, it is better for weight loss if the smallest meal of the day is eaten at night, because that is when your activity level is at its lowest and your basal metabolic rate starts to drop. I've seen people lose weight merely by shifting their meals, eating a larger meal at noon and a smaller meal at night, yet keeping the total calories the same.

But, unfortunately, custom prevails, and in our country the accepted procedure is eating a large evening meal. Most people do not want to give that up.

Whether you eat dinner at 6, 8, or 10 P.M. makes very little difference in the fat-burning sense. Of much greater importance is the total quantity of food you eat. Lighter evening meals facilitate weight loss, heavier evening meals retard it, and the specific evening hour you eat doesn't seem to affect it one way or the other.

Eat or Drink 30 to 40 Percent of Total Daily Requirements in Protein

If you're not losing weight when you are dieting, counting your calories, and balancing your feedings, then you might consider my third principle of effective dieting. Eat 30 to 40 percent of your caloric requirements in protein (meat, fish, eggs, cheese, or nonfat milk). As I stated in Chapter 5, protein is the most important food for growing bodies.

Both proteins and carbohydrates give off four calories per gram. There is evidence, however, that the female with a weight problem does not burn carbohydrates effectively for energy. She stores them as fat. This condition is much more severe in the adult than in the teen-ager, but there is a critical carbohydrate level for everyone. The critical carbohydrate level among teens can comfortably accommodate four to five natural sugars and starches a day in a weight loss program, which can include fruit, cereal, breads, and potatoes or rice. However, if you surpass your critical carbohydrate level, you may *not* lose weight even if you've decreased your calories to 1,000 per day and have balanced your feedings.

Protein, on the other hand, has several metabolic advantages. It has a high SDA (Specific Dynamic Action). It requires more energy to break it down. It forces the body to work.

Protein maintains your blood sugar at a lower level. When blood sugar is high, insulin secretion from the pancreas is high. Insulin blocks the burning of fat. Therefore, it is desirable not to overstimulate the secretion of insulin. Protein does not have a significant insulin response.

Unfortunately, the protein that I prefer (animal protein) is usually combined with fat. Fat has nine calories per gram, so you should try to eat the leanest meat and lowest-fat dairy products.

The regular diets that follow will use the principles I have discussed.

Your success depends on your ability to follow instructions, which is the single most important quality in a dieter. Overweight teens like to bend the rules. No matter how lenient I am, my teen-age patients manage to take advantage.

Many teen-age girls come into my office armed with a long list of "Can I have's?" These usually start out very innocently: "Can I have salt/ketchup/soy sauce?" After I nod yes, they move into more substantial ground. "Can I have bananas/grapes/pomegranates?" If I say yes to these, then they really become exotic. "Can I have ice milk/smoked oysters/soda crackers?" That's when I call a halt. These foods aren't terribly harmful to a diet when eaten in moderation, but teen-agers stretch the limits of a diet enough without giving them more ammunition.

When do you stop following instructions and decide that a diet program is not working for you? Try two weeks of total compliance before you make any decision.

Commitment

Your diet is the most important thing in your life.

(You and I know that is not true—your good health, your family, and your education are much more important than your diet.)

But you must try to believe that, otherwise your diet will take a back seat to everything, In our society, every legal holiday, vacation, birthday, and big date is a legitimate excuse to stray from a weight-reduction diet. Dieting should be like brushing your teeth. No matter what else is going on in your life, you do it!

Therefore, think: Your diet is the most important thing in your life.

Expectations

Many diets and dieters have been ruined by "Great Expectations" that haven't worked out. Many girls think when they start a diet that the weight will fall off them. They think they will wake up in two weeks and be miraculously thin. Not so.

You didn't gain that weight overnight; chances are it took you a long time. So it will take you a long time to lose it. Average weight loss on a nutritious (not crash) diet ranges somewhere between one to two pounds a week after the larger initial weight loss. (Crash diets are quite different and we will discuss them later.)

If you are not losing at least one pound a week, then you should reevaluate what you are doing. If you are losing a steady two pounds a week, you should be very happy—that is a satisfactory and safe weight loss.

There will be weeks when you won't lose one pound, even though you've dieted faithfully. This is called a plateau and is discussed at length in Chapter 15. Do not become discouraged during this time—wait it out!

Knowledge

The knowledgeable dieter is a successful dieter. That's why I've devoted so much space in this book telling you *why* you lose weight, instead of just telling you *ways* to lose it.

You must also try to distinguish useful information from that which is false and misleading. My daughter saw an ad in her favorite teen magazine for a garment that would "melt away fat." She ran to tell me of this new and miraculous discovery. When I told her the advertisement was a big lie, she was shocked. "How could it be a lie?" she asked. "It's right here in the magazine. Why would anybody write an ad that's a lie, and why would anybody print the ad?"

I told her that she should learn early in life that:

1. Fat doesn't melt away.
2. Most magazines will print any ad, as long as it doesn't advocate the overthrow of the government or something illegal.

I know she didn't believe me, and probably went away thinking that I was jealous because I hadn't discovered a garment that would melt away fat. She was probably partly right—I wish I could discover that machine. But in the meantime, you must be particularly careful not to believe everything you read in advertisements, magazine articles, or even books.

11

Diets for Teens

The Carefree Diet

The first diet in this chapter is a liberal diet that teaches you how to eat sensibly. It is a diet for life and requires only small modifications to change it from a weight loss diet to a weight maintenance diet. It does not give you a dramatic weight loss, but rather a gradual, steady loss of about five to eight pounds per month, which allows your body and your head to readjust to your new habits. I call it the Carefree Diet. It doesn't allow you to eat with total abandon, but it does give you many choices. The Carefree Diet has several advantages.

1. No calorie counting.
2. It takes you "off" sugar.
3. It requires no special cooking.
4. It provides good variety and should appeal to many tastes.
5. There are five distinct eating periods, so eating becomes more formalized.
6. It will show you how much food you can consume without gaining weight, if you choose carefully.
7. It provides essential nutrition.
8. It is low in starch, moderate in fat, and high in protein. (This combination seems to be particularly well-suited to the teen-ager's metabolism.)
9. There's no eating in between meals, so your hands and mind are free to do other things.

Eat as much of the following as you want:

> Lean meat, including chicken, turkey, liver, ham, crisp bacon, and sausages
> Fish (canned and fresh) and seafood
> Cheese
> Eggs
> Cottage cheese
> Plain yogurt
> Salads
> Vegetables (except corn or peas)
> Fresh fruits (except grapes)
> Fruit (canned without sugar)
> Condiments (such as sour pickles, ketchup, Worcestershire sauce, soy sauce, mustard, parsley, watercress)
> Beverages such as tea, coffee, low-calorie soda, water, low-calorie lemonade, tomato juice

You may have measured amounts of the following:

> Skim milk (1 pint daily, not including milk in coffee or tea)
> Butter or margarine (1 ounce)
> Bread (high fiber or thin-sliced high protein, 2 slices) or melba toast (4 slices)
> Plain grain products (1 small helping—for example: 1 cup non-sugared cereal, ½ cup rice, or ½ cup macaroni
> Potato (1 baked)
> Peas or corn (½ cup)

The above food should be eaten at meals only. The following foods should be completely avoided:

> Bread (except as previously mentioned)
> Cookies, cakes, or pastries
> Cereal (except as previously mentioned)
> Gravy
> Candy, ice milk, ice cream, pudding, sweetened yogurt
> Soups made with cream
> Sugar
> Syrups, honey, molasses, jellies
> Chocolate, cocoa
> Sweetened fruit drinks or soda
> Potato chips, peanuts, corn chips, or other packaged snacks

In the Carefree Diet, you plan your own meals, but for those girls who need a day-by-day regime, here is what one week of the Carefree Diet might look like.

Breakfast	*Lunch*	*Supper*
Sunday		
½ cantaloupe; French toast (2 slices); skim milk	Cold chicken; tossed salad; Italian dressing; blueberries; skim milk	Roast beef; oven-browned potatoes; string beans; cucumber salad
Monday		
Orange slices; cereal (1 cup); skim milk	cantaloupe; cottage cheese	Roast turkey; low-calorie cranberry sauce; carrots; salad with cheese dressing; pear
Tuesday		
Banana; poached eggs; 1 slice toast; skim milk	Tuna salad sandwich (1 slice bread); raw vegetables; skim milk	Hamburger (lean); string beans; cole slaw; apple
Wednesday		
Cereal with raisins; skim milk	Ham & cheese sandwich; mustard & pickles; orange	Chicken broth (clear); baked chicken; ½ cup corn; Caesar salad; grapefruit
Thursday		
Orange juice; toasted cheese sandwich (1 slice of bread); skim milk	Turkey sandwich with 1 slice of bread, mustard and lettuce; apple	Omelet (3 eggs) with cheese, onions, and peppers; tomatoes and cucumbers; pineapple (fresh or canned)
Friday		
Cold cereal with sliced bananas; skim milk	Yogurt with fresh fruit and raisins	Tomato juice; fish or seafood (broiled); baked potato (pat of butter); tossed salad; skim milk shake
Saturday		
½ grapefruit; scrambled eggs; crisp bacon; skim milk	Chef's salad with cheese, roast beef, Italian dressing; unbuttered popcorn	Steak; asparagus; tomato & lettuce salad; diet gelatin with fresh fruit; skim milk

*Instructions:*Weigh yourself before you begin your diet and then no more than once a week on the same scale, in the same clothes and at the same time, preferably early in the morning.

You should eat three or four meals a day, but try to eat nothing between meals except celery and low-calorie beverages. If you prefer, you can eat three meals and have two small snacks.

Let's go over the Carefree Diet and talk about some of the foods that you'll be eating.

Meat

Lean meat refers to meat that has been trimmed of all available fat. You may eat ham, pork, or lamb chops, as long as they are relatively fat-free.

Certain meats have high levels of fat that you cannot trim away. These include hamburger, bacon, and sausage. The best way to handle them is to cook them until they are *well done* and to drain the excess grease onto paper towels.

I once met a thin, wiry gentleman who claimed to blot up the grease on all meat—even at fancy restaurants. He said he sometimes became the center of attention while dabbing at steak with a cloth napkin, but he boasted of eliminating 100 to 200 calories in fat and felt that it was worth the attention he attracted.

Those of you who have a microwave oven know how dry bacon can be cooked. It should be eaten crisp and flat. Sausages should be pricked with a fork while cooking to release as much oil as possible.

The fattiest meats are the processed ones like bologna, salami, and liverwurst. These should *not* be included in the diet, not only because their fat content is high, but because their protein content is low.

Poultry

Poultry includes chicken and turkey and can be baked or roasted. If the skin is crisp, you may eat it. You can eat any part of the chicken or turkey except the wings, which have too much fat in relation to protein and are extremely high in calories.

A good low-calorie way to prepare chicken breasts is to remove the skin, brush them with soy sauce or low-calorie salad dressing and then charcoal-broil them. Five to seven minutes per side is adequate.

Overcooking turkey is a common and stubbornly repeated cooking error. By the time the dark meat is done correctly, the turkey breast is often dry and tasteless. The white meat cooks in a relatively short time and, when properly prepared, tastes far superior to the disappointingly dry bird that we encounter on holidays. One of my friends used to think that turkey was *supposed* to come out that way—so dry that you choke on it—hence, the gravy to wash it down. Turkey can be just as succulent and delicious as well-prepared turkey breasts and legs, which can be cooked for the precise, individually-suited amount of time that each one needs.

Also, when you're cooking poultry, don't be afraid to use a meat thermometer; it is a simple way to take the guesswork out of preparation.

Seafood

Seafood, which includes shrimp, lobster, crabmeat, clams, and mussels, is an excellent diet food—low in calories, high in protein, available though slightly expensive.

If you can't afford it, you can always have a scoop of tuna fish salad. Even mixed with regular mayonnaise, it's good for a diet.

While we're on the subject of tuna fish salad, I'd like to talk about the use of mayonnaise. Too many restaurants serve soggy, mayonnaise-ridden fish, egg, or chicken salad, where the predominant flavor is the mayonnaise. Use just enough mayonnaise (or diet mayonnaise, if you don't find the taste objectionable) to bind the ingredients in your salads together. You'll appreciate the meat or fish taste a lot more and get far fewer calories. My butter rule is the same—a little butter should go a long way. Lemon or vinegar is also an excellent seasoning for fish, and the more you use, the less mayonnaise you will want.

Eggs

I love eggs. Although they have a high level of cholesterol, they are low-calorie (between 70 and 80 calories each), high-protein, and inexpensive. They are also versatile. You can have them fried or scrambled for breakfast, in egg salad for lunch (light on the mayonnaise, remember), and as omelets for supper.

A lot of teens say to me, "I'm sick of eggs for breakfast. I can't look at another egg." When I ask them if they have tried egg salad for breakfast, they appear shocked and say, "Egg salad for breakfast? I never thought of that." It tastes particularly good in the summertime when you have it on a piece of melba toast with a slice of fresh tomato. You can have an absolutely delicious breakfast and something a little bit different.

I used to hate eggs. but my grandfather changed that. He ate them every day for breakfast. I used to sit and watch him peel the top half of the shell off a soft-boiled egg, salt the exposed white very lightly, and bite it off, leaving the yolk. Then he would scoop out the rest of the egg with a spoon and pop it into his mouth. It was even more fun to watch him eat fried eggs. My grandmother would always fry them perfectly—the white marvelously firm and the yolk just the right consistency. He would carefully eat the white first, leaving the bare yolk on the plate. Then he would deftly slide his knife under the yolk and transport it to his mouth without spilling a drop. It would disappear in one gulp.

After watching him enjoy eggs so often, I wanted to try them, too, although previously I wouldn't touch them. I never mastered his trick of taking the yolk on a knife without breaking it, but the eggs still tasted good.

Cheese

Cheese is another interesting, versatile food, and a good inexpensive source of protein. But beware of American cheese and processed cheese foods, which are carbohydrate solids flavored with cheese. Real cheese has very little carbohydrate in it because it is made from the curd of the milk, and the milk sugar goes into the liquid portion called whey. As much as I object to processed cheese, sometimes eating it helps you develop a taste for real cheese.

Cheese enhances the flavors of many foods. It's good in scrambled eggs; marvelous melted on top of vegetables; and, of course, we know and love it in a cheeseburger. In fact, many kids get hooked on cheeseburgers before they get hooked on cheese. That's okay—it doesn't matter how you're introduced to cheese as long as you become more adventurous.

The new lower-calorie cheese products, which have been on the market for about a year, are a good addition to any diet. (Remember what I keep saying: whenever you can save calories and get the same taste by going to a substitute or similar food, do it.)

I also suggest that you purchase a cheese slicer. Buy unsliced cheese because it keeps a lot longer. Press the slicer across the top, bear down, and you will have beautiful thin slivers. This will help you appreciate the very delicate flavors of different cheeses.

Have you tried rope cheese? It looks like a big braid of hair, and makes a good, low-calorie nibble. You untwist it, soak it in skim milk for a few hours to take out the salt, and then shred it. One braid yields a big bowl of cheese strands, which you can eat as you would candy. It takes a lot of time and is filling, plus you're getting lots of protein and not much carbohydrate.

Don't eat cheese when it's cold—it's not as flavorful. Always let it warm up to room temperature.

Many kids tell me, "I could eat a tremendous amount of cheese; it would be very bad for me to add it to my diet." Actually, most people who eat cheese don't eat it alone. They eat cheese and crackers, cheese and bread, and so on. The problem is obviously in the crackers and bread. If you eat cheese by itself, you won't eat as much as you think. Cheese is one of the foods that you can take only in limited amounts by itself, but in excessive amounts with carbohydrates. Put it on crackers, and you'll eat far more than you should.

Cottage cheese is a favorite with many teens, and if you like it, it is fairly good diet food. I like the low-fat variety better for diets, altough it doesn't taste very good. The only way you should eat cottage cheese is plain or with raw vegetables. Russian salad (in the recipe section) is a tasty way to prepare this food.

Plain cottage cheese is a satisfactory alternative to an egg in the morning and is an excellent source of protein. It contains about 239 calories per cup if it is creamed and about 80 calories less if uncreamed.

The combination you must avoid is the scoop of cottage cheese with fruit (fresh or canned) and a little date-nut sandwich; they could total enough calories for a day.

Yogurt

Yogurt has had good press; advertising has led us to believe that it is one of nature's perfect foods, helping us live longer and feel better. Companies claim that it contains certain organisms that allow you to digest food better. Many leading nutritionists say that indeed there are certain bacterial organisms in yogurt, but they are not the ones that aid digestion. And as for being a dieter's delight, plain yogurt has more calories than a glass of skim milk and no more nutrition—138 to 180 calories in 8 ounces, compared to 77 calories in skim milk.

Yogurt is fermented milk with a high acid content and thick curd. It was invented in areas of the world with poor sanitation; the fermentation protected fresh milk from contamination. When most of us talk about yogurt, we refer to the fruit-flavored kind, sweetened with preserves, or the equally delicious frozen yogurt, plain or topped with fruit. These treats can easily have 300 calories, and the carbohydrate count is high enough to serve as a whole meal. But, if you have a large appetite, yogurt treats won't fill you up, and they have too many calories for snacks (as many teen-agers use them).

Frozen yogurt is only 140 calories per scoop and acceptable as part of a meal. However, it is no better for you than frozen custard or soft ice cream. The only difference would be in your taste preference.

Plain yogurt is most valuable as a diet tool when mixed with vegetables and fresh fruit or as a substitute for sour cream. A friend of mine recently made a cheesecake using yogurt in place of sour cream and it was delicious.

Yogurt is very versatile and can be used to garnish soup or create meat or seafood salads. One tablespoon of yogurt combined with one tablespoon of mayonnaise gives you a lower-calorie mayonnaise, without the sharpness of pure yogurt.

Milk

Milk is our primary source of calcium, and in the growing stage, we need somewhere between 800 and 1,400 milligrams of calcium a day. (Boys probably require more than girls because their bones are much bigger.) One quart of whole milk supplies 1,000 milligrams of calcium and 30 to 35 grams of protein.

Skimming the fat off milk removes some of the vitamins and minerals, but these are then added back before pasteurization. (We say skim milk is "fortified.") Skimming also changes the flavor, which fat enhances.

If milk is "one of our most precious foods," why can't a diet consist of a quart of regular milk and a vitamin pill with iron? It's too boring and would cause intestinal problems in many people. One crash diet, which has gone in and out of popularity over the years, consists of skim milk and bananas. You drink one quart of skim milk and eat six bananas per day. Nobody ever gets sick on that diet because they get sick *of* it before very long.

The only adults in the animal kingdom who voluntarily drink milk after infancy are cats and humans. Babies are *meant* to drink milk, but more and more people are discovering that too much milk or too many milk products give them abdominal pains and cramps, diarrhea, and a bloated feeling. This is due to the presence of lactose, a milk sugar that requires an enzyme called lactase to break it down in the intestine. ("ase" is a suffix that designates enzymes that break down or change food, making it more digestible.)

Many adults are deficient in lactase. This means that the lactose enters the large intestine in an *undigested* state where it has to be broken down by the putrid bacteria in the large bowel. This gives rise to intestinal difficulties. There is also a rising incidence of allergies to milk protein and reports of calcium kidney stones in some large milk drinkers.

It's probably better to get your calcium requirements in cheese, eggs, and leafy vegetables, and to leave milk drinking to babies. This adult intolerance to milk is nature's way of telling us that it's time to diversify our eating habits and to try new foods. That's why I have limited skim milk in the Carefree Diet to one pint, although increasing it would not endanger your weight loss. Rather than drinking it with meals, I find that milk makes a good high-protein snack that curbs the appetite.

If you like milk and want to drink it, *do not* drink whole milk. Skim milk has all the nutrition and almost none of the fat. If you have been a whole milk drinker and hate the taste of skim, switch over gradually. Start by mixing whole milk with *lowfat* milk; then switch to just lowfat milk; finally, switch over to plain skim.

Salads

Salads can be very neglected by teen-agers. What they consider a salad is usually some tired tomatoes and wilted lettuce. Look at the cooking section and see how exciting salads can be. If you're a lettuce-and-tomato or just a lettuce person, you're missing out on some superb combinations.

I went to a restaurant the other day and had a salad with yellow squash, chopped tomatoes, and Italian dressing. I know you're going to say, "Ugh, that sounds gross," but it tasted terrific and was a nice change.

When I travel, I always take a chance in restaurants and order the special or chef's salad. Most of the time, I am pleasantly surprised by the ingenuity with which people put together raw vegetables. Salads with meat and cheese are not always low in calories, but it would take extremely large amounts of other, higher-calorie foods to fill you up as well.

Vegetables

If you're going to diet, you should investigate different kinds of food, especially low-calorie vegetables.

I ask you to exclude corn, peas, and lima beans from the Carefree Diet, and I know that may break a lot of hearts. Well, if you must eat corn or peas, you can probably have limited amounts of them, perhaps half a cup per day. I make an exception in the fresh corn season when you can substitute corn for meat in one or two meals per week. This is because I'm a very nice person, and the corn season is short. However, you can't eat it with butter.

Check the vegetables on this list that you will eat:

_____ Acorn squash

_____ Asparagus

_____ Bamboo shoots

_____ Bean sprouts

_____ Beets

_____ Bok Choy

_____ Broccoli

_____ Brussels sprouts

_____ Cabbage

_____ Carrots

_____ Cauliflower

_____ Celery

_____ Chick peas

_____ Corn

_____ Dandelion greens

_____ Eggplant

_____ Kidney beans

_____ Lettuce (romaine, iceberg, Bibb, endive, and chicory)

_____ Lima beans

_____ Mushrooms
_____ Okra
_____ Parsnips
_____ Pea pods
_____ Peas
_____ Peppers, green
_____ Peppers, red
_____ Scallions
_____ Spinach
_____ Squash, spaghetti
_____ Squash, yellow
_____ String beans
_____ Tomatoes
_____ Turnips
_____ Zucchini

If you have checked less than half of these, you are missing out on a lot of variety that is not only useful in dieting, but necessary in weight maintenance. Also, many of the vegetables that you eat only raw can be eaten cooked, or vice versa. For example, have you ever tried raw string beans or broiled tomatoes?

Fruit

Everyone thinks that fruit is not fattening and that you can eat as much as you want. I would agree that it's more difficult to gain weight on fruit, but you must remember that it is a form of sugar. Granted, in fruit the sugar is combined with water and fiber so that it is diluted. It is very difficult to eat 6 or 7 apples during the course of an evening, but it would be easy to eat the equivalent quantity of sugar (one piece of cake). Still, I have seen many reducing diets ruined by too much fruit. Although the dieter has not gained weight, she has not lost it either. The tendency to overeat occurs too frequently with small pick-up fruits like grapes, which is why I omit them from the diet (although every time there's a grape boycott, people think I do this for political reasons—which are okay, too). Grapes contain only 3 to 4 calories each, but nobody stops at 10 or 20 grapes. The other smaller fruits, like strawberries or blueberries, are seasonal, so they don't tend to pose much of a problem.

There is a myth that watermelon is fattening, probably because it tastes so sweet. If you took all the water out of watermelon, you would have pure watermelon sugar (which was used during the Civil War). However, since watermelon sugar is diluted by about 300 times its own weight in water, one generous slice won't hurt your diet. One advantage of eating watermelon is that it supplies a lot of fluid, which dieting females rarely get enough of.

I have not specifically eliminated dried fruits from the diet, but remember: they have all the calories of regular fruit, without the water. Hence, they don't fill you up as much and you tend to eat more.

Dried fruits are an extremely nutritious, potassium-rich food. They pack easily in a lunch box and don't have to be refrigerated, but they are *deceptively high* in calories. A mere 2 tablespoons of raisins, for example, are 60 calories. True, raisins are convenient and healthy, and if you stop at one snack pack you won't hurt yourself. But if you're going to eat dried fruit, think of it as fresh fruit: 3 raisins are the equivalent of 3 grapes.

Personally, I dislike canned fruit. All the fiber and most of the water has been cooked out of it. Much of the time, it is soggy and uninteresting. Packing fruits in water spoils their taste and makes them watery. Packing them in syrup spoils their taste and makes them high in calories.

The only time it is acceptable to eat fruit canned in water is when you're ill with a sore throat, upset stomach, or diarrhea. Canned fruit is easier to swallow and less likely to aggravate intestinal problems.

When you eat canned fruit, you deprive yourself of good taste, chewing, and satisfaction of hunger, but you get the same amount of calories. One exception is canned pineapple: one slice is only 39 calories, so it is a relatively safe dessert.

As much as I disapprove of fresh fruit as a free nibble food, it is far better than foods made with refined sugar and flour. Often the "smarts" of dieting involves selecting the food that will do you the least harm.

Condiments

Condiments are seasonings that you add to your food to make it taste better. They include ketchup, mustard, soy sauce, teriyaki sauce, Worcestershire sauce, steak sauce, chili, and horseradish.

Ketchup has a lot of sugar, but as most people use it in small quantities, it's not a problem.

However, I had one patient, a male, who mysteriously stopped losing weight when I told him that he could have ketchup. He claimed he was following the diet perfectly, but when I quizzed him about his use of ketchup, he grinned guiltily. "I love ketchup," he said. "You might say that I put food under my ketchup rather than ketchup on top of my food."

Needless to say, that is *not* how to use condiments. They should *enhance* food, not replace it.

Onions can be used as a condiment. They contain a considerable amount of sugar, but in limited quantities are no problem. Add chopped onion to your salad or your hamburger. I don't even object to onions sautéed in a small amount of butter occasionally to dress up a steak. But don't eat stewed onions.

Mustard is a great flavor enhancer. In small quantities you can even use hot, sweet mustard that contains sugar. It tastes especially good on turkey, hamburger, and shrimp. A combination of mustard and ketchup is interesting on hamburgers. Mustard is excellent mixed with deviled eggs, or as the main flavoring for a vegetable dip (combined with yogurt and diet mayonnaise). This kind of dip is relatively low in calories and does not have to be restricted to party use.

I find dill pickles a marvelous addition to a diet, although many of my patients worry about the high salt content. There's something in medicine called "risk-benefit ratio," which means you've got to weigh the benefits of a treatment against the risks and then decide if the risk is worth it. I think that the risk of getting too much salt from a pickle is insignificant when weighed against the benefits.

Dill pickles seem to curb your appetite, and when you put something that sour into your mouth, you don't have as much of a craving for sweets. The next time you eat a pickle, think about whether you really want that piece of chocolate: "chocolate and pickles, yumm…" Pickles are low in calories (15 to 25 depending on the size), require a lot of chewing, and most teen-agers enjoy them. Maybe I'll start a rumor that dill pickles cut or burn away fat—and start a new fad diet.

Beverages

On a diet or off, most girls don't drink enough water. That's because they don't enjoy continually running to the bathroom; and the snide remark, "I know where you are going," still embarrasses them.

They also cling to the idea that water bloats them. Actually, there is some truth in this. Although water is a good diuretic (that is to say, it increases urinary output), females only excrete 60 percent of what they drink. If you drink 10 glasses of water a day, your body will excrete 6 and retain 4. One solution is to lie down several times in the course of the day. This way, water will be mobilized into the kidneys and you will excrete it.

Usually, girls don't take naps in the afternoon. The first time they lie down is at night, and the water is excreted the following morning. This means that the time to measure a female's most accurate weight is early in the morning, after excretion. Later in the day the scale weight will not reflect true fat volume. (Even 2 glasses of skim milk could make the scale go up.)

Why is it important to drink a lot of water on a diet? Because when you diet, you break down a lot of fat and create a lot of waste. The faster you flush these waste products out of your system, the better you will feel. But don't drink ridiculous amounts of water. You can drink 4 glasses of water per day and make up the remainder of your fluid requirements with milk, tomato juice, and diet soda.

Diet soda is controversial at the moment. As of this writing, diet soda with saccharine is still on the market. Scientists have found a connection between saccharine and bladder cancer in animals, and it may not be around much longer. Under no circumstances should you drink regular soda when trying to lose or maintain weight. Try club soda, natural spring water, or iced tea.

I was once on a television show with a very pompous nutritionist, and when the subjects of saccharine, artificial sweeteners, and diet soda came up, she said, "I don't know what gives diabetics the idea that they deserve something sweet." She also said, "Diet soda never kept anybody thin if they didn't want to be thin."

Well, yes ... yes, that's true. I don't think that diet soda *makes* people thin, and perhaps it doesn't keep them thin, but it gives some people a great deal of enjoyment without the nagging guilt feelings they usually have when they put something sweet in their mouths. Nor does it activate any sugar-triggering mechanism in the bloodstream. Often when you desire something sweet, a glass of diet soda is very satisfying and doesn't lead to eating more carbohydrates. In that way, I find it extremely useful.

What about tomato juice? Most teen-agers don't like it, but one of the most helpful things that you could do for yourself would be to acquire a taste for it. Not only is it refreshing, filling, and inexpensive, but it is available almost everywhere. If there's nothing else in the vending machine that you can get, there is usually a can of tomato juice. If there's no other drink in a cocktail lounge, there's always a Bloody Mary, and you can get it without the alcohol; the spicy tomato flavor is very appealing.

Soup

I haven't mentioned soup as a diet food because I don't believe it's very useful. The soup companies would like you to believe that a bowl of soup is a nutritious lunch, and it is when combined with a sandwich or fruit. By itself, however, most uncreamed soup is 100 to 150 calories per serving. Protein values of most labeled chicken or beef soups are painfully low. You get a lot of starch, fat, and salt, but not very much protein.

And soup doesn't last very long in your stomach; if you eat nothing else, you will be hungry an hour later. If you eat it with a sandwich and fruit, you're getting too many calories. If you eat it as a first course, it fills you up, and you'll eat less of the more nutritious main course.

Soup can be valuable as a temporary filler for the person who comes home starving at 4:30 in the afternoon. It is essential that you choose a soup that is low in calories; bouillon or consommé are the ideal choices. They have very few calories and can take the edge off hunger. Vegetable, chicken, or beef bouillon can be used. There are also certain homemade soups (see recipes in Chapter 21) that have no fat and are good for dieting. These vegetable soups coupled with a protein source like cheese, eggs, and a salad give you a satisfying, low-calorie meal.

If you're using a meat-base soup that's homemade, you must refrigerate it overnight and skim off the fat before it is heated and eaten.

If you love soup, eat it as a first course and give up fruit for dessert. While you're not getting the same nutrients, particularly the vitamins, and are getting more salt (which I don't worry about), it's still a reasonable exchange, calorie-wise.

Hot Dogs

I do not include hot dogs in the meat protein section because they are not uniform in preparation. Some brands have large amounts of fat and filler; others are pure meat (Kosher hot dogs are all beef). The difference in calories is vast, ranging from 120 to 180.

Many of my patients adore hot dogs and prefer them to most other meats. I allow you to eat two or three twice a week in place of meat.

The problem with these processed meats is that the fat is beautifully disguised; most people don't even realize it's there. That plump, juicy look unfortunately comes from the same thing that makes you look plump and juicy—fat. One way to get rid of some of it is to boil processed meats instead of grilling them. You can get an idea of how much fat there is in a product from the little blobs of grease that rise to the top of the water.

The Dependable Diet for Active Teens

There are many diets that are very useful for teen-agers. I divide them into diets for the active and inactive teen. How do you know whether you are active or inactive? Answer these questions as a very rough guide:

1. Do you participate in a school sport other than gym?
2. Do you walk at least one mile a day in addition to the walking you must do?
3. Would you rather play soccer or tennis than read a book or watch TV?
4. Would you rather run than bowl?

If you answer yes to three out of these four questions, you definitely qualify for the Dependable Diet for active teens. If you answer yes to two of them, you should try it.

Breakfast	Juice or fruit; 2 eggs fried or broiled; 1 slice toast or ½ bagel or ½ English muffin; nonfat milk *or* Juice or fruit; hot or cold cereal, one tsp. sugar; nonfat skim milk

Lunch Sandwich: 2 slices of bread or a roll; filling: 4 oz. roast beef , chicken, or tuna fish; mayonnaise, lettuce, tomato, mustard, ketchup; dessert: any fresh fruit, except grapes

Snacks Skim milk with hard-boiled egg or raw vegetable with 1 oz. hard cheese

Supper Any kind of lean meat or fish, broiled (all you can eat); salad (all you can eat) oil and vinegar dressing; cooked vegetable (all you can eat) except corn and peas, which are limited to ½ cup; fresh fruit, one piece (you may save this for later)

Snacks Baked potato or fresh fruit

Free Foods Dill pickles, raw vegetables, diet gelatin

Onions may be used as a condiment.

Canned fruit in its own juice can be substituted for fresh fruit, but remember, it won't fill you up as much and you will tend to eat more.

Diet dressing can always be used instead of oil and vinegar, and plain lemon juice would be just great.

Remember, fruit is not a free food although it's the best carbohydrate that you can eat. Too much will stop your weight loss.

You may drink decaffeinated coffee, herb tea, diet soda, tomato juice, or nonfat milk.

The Dependable Diet is essentially my "high-calorie, weight-loss diet," which was my original diet for all teen-agers. It worked beautifully for teen-age boys, but unless teen-age girls were extremely active, it didn't work as well.

I got the idea of using a baked potato for a snack when I was sitting in a coffee shop in Florida, watching a group of girls. Most of them ordered the usual snacks from soda to cake. One girl loudly announced that she was on a diet and ordered a baked potato. I was amazed.

When the potato came, I watched her eat it. It took a long time. In fact, she was still eating after her friends had finished their desserts. She seemed to be chewing a great deal more and getting a lot more satisfaction. Most important, she didn't feel sorry for herself because she was dieting. If she had been munching on lettuce leaves or drinking iced tea, she would have felt like a martyr.

Baked potatoes make a lot of sense as a snack. They're filling, tasty, simple, and require some time to prepare, which always gives you time to ask yourself if you really want it. If you decide between the preparation time and the eating that you don't want it, you can always wrap it in tinfoil and reheat it later.

Another unique way to use a baked potato on a diet was brought to my attention by a thin friend as we were dining in a local fast-food house. She ordered a scoop of cottage cheese and a baked potato. As she mashed the baked potato and mixed the cottage cheese, she explained to me that the cottage cheese supplied the protein, and the potato substituted for her fruit. This kind of lunch, she said, suited her. It was easy to maintain her weight, cut down on her meat intake, and still feel full. She was eating only 230 calories in a diet rich in protein, calcium, and vitamins. That was a real bargain.

Dial-a-Diet

Sometimes after a long day at school you don't have the energy or imagination to plan meals with a lot of variety. "Dial-a-Diet" gives you that variety, with enough suggestions to keep you from getting too bored and giving you some ideas about the kinds of combinations that you can create. Any one of these breakfasts, lunches, or suppers can be mixed and matched. If you refuse to eat breakfast, here are three quick and easy "nonbreakfasts."

1. 4 oz. orange juice and 8 oz. skim milk
2. A granola bar and skim milk
3. Fruit and skim milk

To construct a dial, find an old spinner from one of your board games, or use a toothpick with one end squared off. Place it in the center of the dial and spin. Do this the night before and spin all three meals.

Breakfast

---

nonsweetened cereal
fresh fruit
skim milk

2 eggs, 2 ozs. orange
juice,
high fiber toast
nonfat milk

cottage cheese and
ketchup
melba toast

Dial-a-Diet

2 oz. juice
high protein bread
one slice of cheese

cottage cheese with
cinnamon
and one teaspoon sugar
melba toast

egg salad
juice

Lunch

---

sandwich: 2 slices of bread,
or 1 roll or 1 bagel;
beef, chicken, turkey
tuna or cheese; mustard, ketchup

baked potato
1 cup cottage cheese
raw vegetables

tuna salad plate
fresh raw vegetables
fresh fruit

4 oz. hamburger or 2
hot dogs (no bun)
salad, 1 tbsp. dressing
fresh fruit

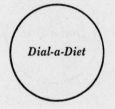

Dial-a-Diet

1 cup of soup
(no noodles or rice)
cold chicken or tuna
fresh fruit, salad

cheese omelet
small salad
fresh fruit

cheese slices on
highfiber bread;
1 orange

chef's salad with meat,
cheese, and eggs; 2 tbsp.
diet salad dressing

Supper

---

4 or 8 or 12 oz. beef, chicken,
turkey, fish, lamb, or veal
salad with diet dressing
fresh fruit

3-egg omelet
asparagus and zucchini
diet gelatin with
fresh fruit

8 oz. fish, chicken,
veal or turkey
1 cup rice with tomato sauce
salad (apple, celery, and
diet mayonnaise)

6 oz. beef
salad, diet dressing
cooked vegetable
fresh fruit

Dial-a-Diet

salad niçoise,
rye crisp, pear

vegetable plate
(string beans, carrots,
broccoli, beets)
oatmeal cookies (2)

1 bowl of soup
(no noodles or rice)
4 oz. any protein
(meat, fish, cheese)
large salad (oil and vinegar)
string beans

In addition to 3 meals, you may have a snack:

Active teens: baked potatoes or fresh fruit, melba toast
All teens: hard-boiled eggs, 1 or 2 oz. cheese,
melba toast, and nonfat milk

The Double Diet

If you place yourself in the category of the inactive teen-ager, this Double Diet is a more appropriate diet for you (incidentally, teen-agers on the pill, or who have had pregnancies or surgery, might do better on this diet).

It is called the Double Diet because for supper you simply double the amount of food you had for lunch.

Breakfast	2 oz. orange juice; 2 eggs; 1 slice of melba toast or ½ grapefruit; 1 cup dry cereal, Skim milk (no sugar)
Lunch	4 oz. meat or fish (diet mayonnaise may be used with tuna fish) 1 cup of salad with diet dressing or cooked vegetables (no corn or peas) 1 fresh fruit
Supper	You may have the same things as at lunch but double the amounts
Snack	½ oz. hard cheese or 1 hard-boiled egg Raw vegetables
Free Foods	Raw vegetables, dill pickles, diet gelatin

There is nothing difficult or unpleasant about the Dependable Diet or the Double Diet. No one says that you must eat fish or drink milk if you hate them, but you must follow the general plan of the diet. Discipline is the principle of dieting; specific substitutions can be worked out (up to a point).

Calorie-Counting Diets

You must have noticed that in the preceding diets, I have not actually counted calories! However, there are certain parents who insist on relative calorie counts for teen-age dieting. Therefore, I have a group of menus that illustrate distinct levels of calories. This is merely to give you an idea of the amount of food it takes to make up a certain number of calories. You might like to go on one of these diets for a week and see how much you lose, given a known amount of calories.

The following are about 900-calorie, balanced-deficit diets. (Balanced-deficit diets are diets that are balanced but reduced in calories. They are not high-protein, low-carbohydrate, or lowfat.)

Day 1

Breakfast ½ grapefruit; ½ English muffin; 1 cup lowfat frosted chocolate drink

Lunch 1 cup vegetable soup; 2 oz. turkey, thin bread (turkey sandwich) lettuce, tomato, mustard; diet soda

Supper 4 oz. broiled fish with margarine; 1 cup broccoli spears, cucumber, sliced tomato, and vinegar; fresh fruit

Day 2

Breakfast 4 oz. orange juice; 1 fried egg; 1 slice melba toast with diet jelly; 8 oz. skim milk

Lunch 4 oz. lowfat cottage cheese; 1 small tomato, sliced; 1 small cucumber, zucchini; ½ cup bean sprouts with diet dressing; 1 slice melba toast

Supper 1 cup consommé; Italian meatballs with tomato sauce; ½ cup rice; garden salad with diet French dressing; 1 cup green beans; ½ cup whipped diet gelatin dessert

Day 3

Breakfast 4 oz. orange juice; 1 cup puffed rice; 1 cup skim milk

Lunch 3 ¾ oz. water-packed tuna with lemon and oregano, tomato, lettuce, and green pepper; 2 crisp rye crackers

Supper Grilled Cheddar cheese sandwich on 1 slice bread with sliced tomato; mixed green salad with diet dressing; fresh blueberries

Day 4

Breakfast 2-egg omelet made with 1 tsp. margarine; 1 slice melba toast; 4 oz. plain yogurt, mixed with 1 tsp. honey or vanilla

Lunch Lean hamburger patty (3 oz.) with a dill pickle; garden salad with 1 tbsp. diet dressing; 1 fresh orange

Supper Broiled chicken breast with seasoned salt; 1 cup green beans, cooked; lemon wedge with tomato slice and diet dressing; 1 fresh pear

Day 5

Breakfast 4 oz. tomato juice; 1 hard-cooked egg; 1 slice thin whole wheat bread; 1 tsp. diet jelly; 1 low-calorie frosted vanilla drink

Lunch 1 cup chicken egg-drop soup; 3 oz. salmon salad (small can of salmon made into a salad with 1 tsp. diet mayonnaise); celery stuffed into whole tomato; 1 crisp rye cracker; 8 oz. skim milk

Supper 4 oz. lean baked ham; 6 asparagus with sesame seeds/ lemon wedge with diet dressing; diet applesauce; skim milk

Day 6

Breakfast 1 cup (fresh or frozen) unsweetened strawberries; 1 slice French toast made with bread, skim milk, 1 egg, and a pinch of vanilla; 1 cup skim milk

Lunch 1 cup beef bouillon; 1 pita bread filled with chopped cheese, alfalfa sprouts, tomato, onion, with 1 tbsp. taco sauce; diet soda

Supper 4 oz. lean roast beef; 1 baked potato; garden salad with 1 tbsp. diet dressing; ½ cup pineapple tidbits

Day 7

Breakfast 1 tangerine; Western omelet with 2 eggs, onion, green pepper, mushrooms, and Cheddar cheese; 2 slices melba toast; 8 oz. skim milk

Lunch 1 tbsp. peanut butter, 1 tsp. diet jelly, and 1 slice thin bread; 3 celery sticks, carrot sticks; 1 medium size fresh apple; diet soda

Supper 5 oz. broiled scallops with margarine, marinated in lemon juice, garlic, parsley, teriyaki sauce; fresh spinach salad made with 1 cup spinach, bean sprouts, diet dressing; 1 cup parsleyed carrots; diet gelatin dessert

The following are about 1,400-calorie, balanced-deficit diets.

Day 1

Breakfast 4 oz. orange juice; 2 slices French toast, thin bread, diet syrup, 1 tsp. diet margarine; 2 slices crisp bacon; low-calorie frosted vanilla drink

Lunch   2 hot dogs, 1 bun with mustard, 1 cup sauerkraut; 1 medium tangerine

Supper   ½ barbecued chicken, ¼ cup barbecue sauce; 1 baked potato; 1 cup green beans; lettuce salad with diet dressing; lime diet gelatin dessert

Day 2

Breakfast   8 oz. plain yogurt with 1 banana sliced into it

Lunch   3 oz. lean roast beef on 2 slices thin whole wheat bread; sliced tomatoes, alfalfa sprouts and diet mayonnaise; 1 tangelo; skim milk

Supper   4 oz. tomato juice with a lemon twist; cheese and mushroom omelet with 3 eggs, 1 oz. lowfat cheese, taco sauce, 1 tsp. diet margarine (for frying); tossed salad with diet dressing; ½ cup ice milk

Day 3

Breakfast   ½ grapefruit; 1 scrambled egg/1 tsp. imitation bacon bits; 1 slice thin whole wheat toast; 2 tsp. diet margarine/diet jelly; 8 oz. skim milk

Lunch   Open-faced cheeseburger (3 oz. meat/1 oz. cheese/½ roll/lettuce/ tomato); dill pickle; 10 French fries/ketchup; fresh medium apple; diet soda

Supper   4 oz. lean pork chops marinated in teriyaki sauce; ½ cup noodles/1 tsp. caraway seeds; spinach/cherry tomato salad/2 tbsp. diet dressing; ½ cup whipped lime diet gelatin dessert; 8 oz. low-calorie vanilla frothy

Day 4

Breakfast   4 oz. orange juice; ¾ cup cornflakes/2 tbsp. wheat germ/artificial sweetener; 8 oz. skim milk

Lunch   Chef salad/lettuce/tomato/cucumber/green olives and 2 oz. lowfat cheese/1 oz. ham, turkey, or roast beef/2 tbsp. diet dressing; 2 bread sticks; ¼ cantaloupe; diet soda

Supper   Beef consommé; 4 oz. roast turkey *au jus*; ½ cup stuffing; 1 cup broccoli/1 tsp. diet margarine; shredded lettuce/diet dressing; plain pound cake square (3 x 3); 8 oz. low-calorie milk frothy

Day 5

Breakfast 1 tangerine; 1 hard-cooked egg; 8 oz. low-calorie vanilla frothy

Lunch 3 oz. ham/1 oz. Swiss cheese/lettuce/tomato/mustard; 2 slices thin diet bread; 8 oz. skim milk

Supper 1 cup cooked spaghetti/4 oz. meat sauce/1 tsp. Parmesan cheese; 1 slice garlic bread/1 tsp. diet margarine/pressed garlic; tossed salad/2 tbsp. diet Italian dressing; ½ cup minted pineapple chunks; diet soda

Day 6

Breakfast 4 oz. orange juice; 1 slice thin bread/2 slices lowfat American cheese/mustard; 8 oz. skim milk

Lunch 3 oz. shrimp salad/1 tbsp. diet mayonnaise/2 tsp. minced celery; 1 slice thin bread; 6 black olives; 1 medium fresh pear; 8 oz. skim milk

Supper 4 oz. lean sirloin steak smothered with mushrooms; 1 medium baked potato/2 tbsp. plain yogurt or diet sour cream and chives; 1 cup wax beans; 1 cup red cabbage slaw/1 tsp. oil and vinegar; ½ cup homemade applesauce/artificial sweetener/cinnamon

Day 7

Breakfast 1 fried egg/1 slice American cheese/1 slice Canadian bacon/1 toasted English muffin; 8 oz. skim milk

Lunch 3 oz. tuna fish salad/2 slices bread/1 tbsp. minced green pepper/1 tbsp. diet mayonnaise; 2 slices thin rye bread; 3 celery sticks/3 carrot sticks; ½ fresh grapefruit/artificial sweetener; diet soda

Supper 4 oz. orange juice; lasagna (4″ x 3″ x 2″ square); spinach salad/bean sprouts/mushrooms/2 tbsp. diet dressing; whipped diet gelatin dessert; low-calorie chocolate frothy

12

The Big Crash

Everybody in school envied Susan; she was beautiful in the dark-haired, almond-eyed manner of a young Elizabeth Taylor, and she went out with Todd—that gorgeous blond hunk of class president and football captain. *Beautiful people.*

Or beautiful until Susan began putting on weight, just a little at a time, a chocolate bar's worth here, a banquet's worth there. It didn't really show until Susan caught mononucleosis during her junior year and spent six weeks in bed. To keep up Susan's strength, her mother fed her constantly.

When Susan emerged from her convalescence, she had gained so much weight that she could barely get into her clothes. So her mother bought her jeans a size larger, and she hid her new chubbiness under baggy, tent-sized shirts.

Todd, who had been very kind about Susan's weight, began to get disgusted with the way she looked. He couldn't give her those sparkling, blue-eyed stares anymore; he found himself looking away more and more often. So Todd lost his sparkle, and Susan didn't look so pretty with jowls and a double chin and fat, round cheeks that squashed her violet eyes.

But Todd really liked Susan and tried to hide his embarrassment when he was with her in public. Occasionally he would let a little remark slip like, "Hey, maybe you shouldn't eat so much," or "Gee, Susan, do you really need that second piece of cake?"

The junior prom was coming up in a few weeks—the shimmering highlight of high school for girls like Susan, and even rather nice for guys like Todd, who might trade it for the chance to score another winning touchdown in the big game, but who still loved it when everybody envied his twinkling, tuxedoed manliness and beautiful—well, sort of—girl friend.

Susan began to look for a prom gown. She knew what she wanted; she had been picturing it for years: a very pale pink or lavender gown that would set off her black hair and violet eyes. Maybe it would be strapless or have spaghetti straps or a ruffle around the shoulders, fitted to the hips and falling loosely in a flare of organdy. She had magical, tantalizing visions of she and Todd dancing through the night, whirling around the decorated gym while other couples gazed in speechless admiration.

In the dress store, Susan started poking around her usual sizes 6 and 8, until a smartly-dressed saleslady approached her. "May I help you, dear?" asked the woman, sweetly. "I think you're in the wrong size."

"But I always wear this size," protested Susan.

The woman smiled even more sweetly and said, "Perhaps we can interest you in something in the 12s or 14s."

Susan was furious, anguished. She stomped out and vowed never to shop in that store again. She went to a store that she didn't like as much, and this time began looking at size 10 (she didn't want the saleslady to make any cracks). But she could not help thinking that the styles looked cuter when they were smaller, so she picked up the same gown in three different sizes and scurried into the dressing room.

The size 6 was a joke. It wouldn't even fit over the tops of her arms. With considerable straining she managed to pull the size 8 over her, but the zipper gaped so much that she was afraid the dress would come apart when she breathed. The size 10 was so tight that she could barely move, but at least she could take small breaths. "Be thankful for small blessings," she thought.

At this point came a little knock from the saleslady. "Need any help in there?" she called cheerfully.

"Thank you, no," snapped Susan, acidly. "I'm just fine."

She carefully tugged off the 10, slipped on her jeans and shirt, and replaced the three dresses on their racks. She paused. Out of the corner of her eye she saw a rack of 12s. No, not that, never that! a 12?

It fit. Somehow her body had ballooned into a size 12. She stared painfully into the mirror. Oh no, she thought, this can't be me. This can't be *me*! Where the top of the dress met her skin, where it should have been nice and smooth and sexy, little bulges of fat crept out. In the back she could see the lumps. Where her stomach should have been flat was a roll of flab, and the dress had bunched up around the tops of her hips. Yes, it was the perfect dress, but she looked *terrible*.

Susan debated. Should she buy the dress and go on a diet? Should she wait until a week before the prom and buy a smaller size? Then she had an idea....

Finally it was prom night. Scarcely able to suppress her excitement, Susan slipped the dress over her body. She looked beautiful: her skin was smooth; there were no little lumps of fat; and her stomach was flat. Her cheeks had color and her eyes sparkled. She had fixed her hair in a breathtaking new way, brushed back and held with a lavender comb that matched her dress.

At the prom, all heads turned as Todd led his beautiful girl friend onto the dance floor, his blue eyes sparkling as he took her into his strong arms. She thought she had never felt such ecstasy. She saw the colored lights merge as he spun her around, the voices of the couples fading into a hum, and the music growing distant....

With effort, Susan opened her eyes. A mob of people was standing over her. She was on a sofa. She closed her eyes, and the blackness began to spin into dizzying patterns of light. She could hear her name called, over and over, and she managed to get one more look at Todd. His eyes no longer sparkled.

Do you know why Susan passed out on the dance floor?

Two weeks earlier, she had decided to buy the size 10 gown. To go from a 12 to a 10, Susan knew she had to lose at least 16 pounds, a large amount of weight for a girl who had only dieted once before, losing between three and four pounds. The diet she had picked is a teen favorite:

Susan's Crash Diet _____

Breakfast	Nothing
Lunch	Some juice
Supper	Some more juice

How did her family and Todd let her get away with this ridiculous routine? When the family was having supper, Susan always claimed to be studying. "I'll come down and eat it later," she would tell them, at which time she would dump her food into the garbage disposal. When Todd took her out for sodas after school, Susan would explain that she had eaten a big lunch, and would chew sugarless gum and drink a glass of water .

At the end of two weeks, Susan had lost an enormous 16 pounds. But she didn't feel so well. When she rose quickly she felt very dizzy, but at least her stomach had stopped hurting from hunger and had flattened out nicely. Her cheeks even had that interesting sunken-cheeked look of a model. She overcame her weakness by thinking about the prom.

If Todd had known about her "diet," he would have been furious. As a sportsperson, he knew that the way to diet isn't to starve yourself, that the body needs certain nutrients to survive. It requires protein, vitamins, and minerals, and a certain amount of carbohydrate. Susan had depleted her system of everything it needed.

Susan never got back to the dance floor. Todd took her home, where her family threatened to take her to the hospital unless she told them what was wrong. She confessed, and her mother forced her to eat a large dinner. The next day Susan stepped on the scale and discovered she had gained six pounds. Within 10 days she gained back all her weight. The starving had been for nothing.

What should Susan have done? She should have bought the size 12 gown and gone on a more sensible crash diet. She should have exercised regularly to tighten up some of the muscles that had become flabby from lying in bed. If the strenuous exercise proved impossible for her, she should have walked rapidly around her house several times a day. She would have felt much better and could have continued to diet sensibly after the prom was over. Instead, she was force-fed by alarmed parents.

Susan's stunt was nothing new, part of an old misconception about how to eat: all or nothing. This is why most dieters never keep their weight off. They don't understand that in between the two extremes is a safe, sensible way of losing or maintaining weight.

Crash and Safe Landing

I used to disapprove of crash diets because they teach the dieter nothing about eating, but I have since softened my opinion. Crash diets are okay as long as you understand *why* you're losing weight. There is nothing magical about them; they are a fast, effective way to lose weight in an emergency.

Say the prom is two weeks off. Like Susan, you slide into your dress and look lumpy. Your face is pale and puffy. You've been hitting the cookie jar and the scale says you weigh six or seven pounds too much. It all went to your middle and your hips; your stomach keeps popping out. Time is of the essence. You don't have a severe weight problem, but you've always wanted to be a little thinner, to look trim in your jeans. For someone like you, a crash diet can be safe, gratifying, and even fun. If you have more than 15 pounds to lose, avoid the crash because you'll never lose *all* the weight and will end up frustrated.

A crash diet is drastically lower in calories than regular diets because it's designed for rapid weight loss. It's low in sugars and starches because they hold water and you want to have a big water loss. It should be monotonous so you don't overeat (you get tired of the same food). A crash diet should be simple, sane, and short (two weeks maximum).

In the crash diet, daily intake should not exceed 1,000 calories. The problem is how to look good, feel good, fill yourself up, and get the proper nutrition from those 1,000 calories. As long as it meets minimum daily requirements for good health, a crash diet can consist of anything you want. Those requirements are:

Protein: At least 6 oz. of meat or fish
Calcium: One pint of nonfat milk
Potassium: Plenty of green leafy vegetables, oranges
Vitamins: One multivitamin pill
Bulk: Salad, raw vegetables

Crashes in hot weather require more potassium-rich foods than in cold weather because you lose a lot more fluids when you sweat.

How can you fill yourself up on a crash diet? That's the point of eating the same food—you get bored with it. If you're bored with food, you're less likely to eat too much of it. (In one experiment, overweight people were fed a vanilla liquid-diet supplement that tasted so bland that they ate less than people of normal weight.) Don't use any of the things that make food a little tastier—no ketchup, salad dressings, spices—and very little salt. Eat no favorite fruits like apples or bananas.

One of the biggest problems in crash dieting is that after two or three days, the dieter begins to feel weak or light-headed and many misinterpret this feeling as a need for food. But as long as you're protecting your body protein, your system gets plenty of nutrition by feeding off your excess fat. This, of course, is true of both regular and crash diets. Your weakness comes from loss of water and occasionally from low blood sugar.

Fifty to sixty percent of your initial weight loss will always be water. Where does this water weight come from?

1. *The liver:* Sugar stored in the liver holds four times its weight in water. This sugar is used up early in dieting, and the water is excreted through the urine.
2. *Fat.* Fat is 20 percent water, which you release when you burn calories.
3. *Between the cells.* Extracellular water is normal. However, it can be increased by high carbohydrate diets, certain hormone levels, and salt intake. When any of these variables are decreased, you lose the excess water.

The problem with losing all that water is that it makes you feel dry. Along with the water you lose potassium, a mineral necessary for muscle strength, and its loss can make you feel tired. In addition, by decreasing your food supply, your blood sugar drops because there's no constant supply of carbohydrates for fast energy.

One of the tricks in crash dieting is to have a very low-calorie, high-protein snack between meals. This way you never go for too long without food. Another trick is to eat lots of low-calorie, high-potassium foods like tomatoes, spinach, Brussels sprouts, cabbage, or the more popular, but high-calorie, orange.

I use several crash diets, but my sentimental favorite, the Sunshine Diet, is one that I discussed in my last book. I made this up one day when a girl came into my office and demanded something "different." She didn't want anything complicated and wanted to lose ten pounds in two weeks. It was a beautiful, sunny day outside, so I looked out the window and said, "I have just the diet for you—the Sunshine Diet!" It was terribly kooky, but she lost ten pounds and felt wonderful.

Crash No. 1—The Sunshine Diet

Breakfast   1 orange; 1 glass skim milk (8 oz.); 1 multivitamin pill
This should appeal to girls who don't want to sit down and eat a big breakfast. I prefer 1 orange to a glass of juice because it contains roughage—fiber and bulk.

Lunch	1 orange; 1 glass skim milk (8 oz.); 1 hamburger patty (3 oz.) (Yes, I said hamburger patty. Cook it at home and bring it to school cold. If you don't like cold hamburger, you can substitute a 3-oz. cube steak for a hamburger patty. If you hate beef, substitute a small chicken breast.)
After-school snack	1 hard-boiled egg *or* 1 oz. American cheese; 1 glass skim milk (4 oz.)
Supper	1 orange; 1 glass skim milk (8 oz.); 2 hamburger patties (3 oz. each); 1 large salad made with any raw vegetable, with vinegar or lemon juice as a dressing
Late-evening snack	1 glass skim milk (4 oz.) *or* 1 glass tomato juice *or* 1 hard-boiled egg
Free liquids	Water; diet soda; club soda; tea or coffee
Snack	Celery

Why do you lose a lot of weight on this diet? I've reduced your caloric intake drastically, but I've given you sufficient protein (hamburger), calcium (milk), potassium and bulk (oranges), and vitamins. Your carbohydrate intake is reduced a great deal, so you will have a rather large water loss the first week. Notice how much you run to the bathroom.

To avoid gaining all your weight back the week after the Sunshine Diet, stick to the same format but add more food. For breakfast, add 1 cup of nonsugared cereal. For lunch, add a salad with diet dressing. For supper, add an unlimited amount of cooked vegetables (but no corn or peas). The following week you can resume normal eating, but don't have any sweet desserts.

Crash Diet No. 2

Breakfast	2 eggs, cooked any way with 1 tsp. butter; ½ grapefruit
Midmorning	Tomato juice; skim or nonfat milk
Lunch	Plain tuna fish on a plate with 1 orange; celery; skim milk *or* lowfat cottage cheese

After school   ½ banana skim or nonfat milk

Supper   Chicken *or* tuna *or* broiled beef; large salad with diet dressing; ½ grapefruit; skim milk *or* lowfat cottage cheese

Free liquids and between meals   Same as in Sunshine Diet

Stay on this diet for two weeks.

How will you look for the prom? Smashing! Your face won't be puffy, your eyes will be bright, your hair will be lustrous, and you'll fit into that gown again.

And, you won't pass out.

One-Week Crash Dieting

Sometimes it is necessary to go on a one-week instead of a two-week crash. The real trick of the one-week crash isn't to lose the weight, but to keep from gaining it all back the second week. There are two one-week crashes that give you sufficient quantities of protein and adequate weight loss. These are for the girl who is not obese, but has gained a few extra pounds and wants to get ready for the beach, take an unexpected trip, or look her best in a play.

The Crazy Crash

Day 1   Nothing but the following liquids—all you desire (orange juice is the only limited one): 4 oz. orange juice (2 oz. in morning and 2 oz. in afternoon); nonfat milk; tomato juice; decaffeinated coffee; bouillon; consommé; diet gelatin dessert; diet soda; lowfat dairy drink mix.

Day 2   Add 10 oz. lean beef, broiled chicken, or fish (either canned or fresh). This must be divided into at least two feedings.

Day 3   Add 2 large salads with any raw vegetable, using vinegar, lemon juice, or salt and pepper.

Day 4   Add a breakfast: 2 eggs prepared any way; 1 piece melba toast.

Day 5   Add 1 slice of melon or 1 orange.

Day 6   Add 2 oz. hard cheese.

Day 7   Add a fresh fruit.

The first day of this diet is the most difficult because you are drinking your caloric intake. There are several things that you should do to make it more comfortable. You can arrange your liquids as if you are eating a meal. For instance, for breakfast you can have 2 oz. orange juice, a glass of tomato juice, and a glass of skim milk. For lunch you can have tomato-vegetable juice, consommé or bouillon (beef or chicken), diet gelatin, and skim milk. For supper you can have 2 oz. orange juice, beef bouillon, lowfat dairy drink mix and diet gelatin. In between meals you should take either skim milk or tomato juice.

You should have as little caffeine as possible during this particular day because it tends to make you irritable. Therefore, diet drinks should not be cola-flavored, and you should avoid coffee or tea. These should not be added until the third day of the diet.

For protein needs, you should try to drink 1 pint of milk, or chocolate lowfat dairy drink mix that day. Any vegetable that can be eaten raw is permitted in the salad that you add on the third day, even if it is not the usual vegetable for salads—string beans, broccoli, cauliflower, along with the usual lettuce and tomato. If you do not want breakfast on Day 4, you may have your 2 eggs as snacks, one at 10:30 A.M. and the other at 3:30 P.M.

Crash No. 2*

Breakfast 4 oz. nonfat milk; tea or decaffeinated coffee (unlimited) without sugar or cream

Lunch Choose one of the following (broiled or boiled, 3½ oz., only): eye of the round, chicken breast (no skin), filet of sole, shrimp, lobster tails, crabmeat, water-packed tuna fish
Choose an average serving of one vegetable (fresh or cooked): celery, ¼ head of lettuce, 1 tomato, red radishes, cucumbers, spinach, cabbage, 1 green pepper; cooked vegetables include asparagus, cauliflower, spinach, celery, tomatoes, cabbage, mushrooms, string beans
1 piece melba toast
Choose 1 medium orange, medium apple, or small whole grapefruit

Dinner The same four choices as lunch

*HCG diet without the HCG—This was the diet I used when I thought HCG (Human Chorionic Gonadatrophin, a chemical extract from pregnant females) was the answer to overeating. It proved to be a total flop, but the 500-calorie, balanced diet that went with it is occasionally useful.

Note: Tea, coffee, plain water, mineral water, and 16 to 20 oz. of low-calorie soda can be used to make up a minimum of 2 quarts of liquid daily. Salt, pepper, vinegar, dry mustard, garlic, sweet basil, parsley, oregano, and onion can be used for seasoning. The juice of one lemon is allowed daily.

The fruit portions may be eaten with lunch or dinner or at other times, but do not combine the lunch and dinner portions into one meal.

When the week is up, continue for one more day on the diet. Beginning the second day, increase the amount of food by 2 eggs, ½ cup of lowfat cottage cheese, and 1 glass of skim milk a day. Increase melba toast to 2 or 3 slices, breakfast and lunch. Meals now include all various cuts of steak and veal. Continue eating this way for one more week. Then resume normal eating habits, but without refined sugar.

Most two-week crashes are good for 7 to 10 pounds and most one-week crashes, 4 to 6 pounds. Remember, not all of this is fat. Twenty to thirty percent is body water that will be regained rapidly when you start to eat carbohydrates.

13

Vegetarian Diets

Many people used to associate vegetarians exclusively with the "counterculture"; they wore jeans, smoked dope, held leftist views, and had the audacity to reject good old red-blooded American meat for rolled oats.

Today the trend is beginning to reverse—meat and meat-eaters have fallen under suspicion. More and more young people are shunning "cannibalism" and "returning to nature," eating foods that are higher in fiber and lower in saturated fat and cholesterol. Most college campuses now serve vegetarian alternatives at every meal, and as meat prices rise, even traditional American cooks are sampling soy burgers, vegetable quiches, and granola. Besides, by the year 2000, meat may be so scarce and expensive that most of us won't be eating very much of it.

Parents, however, still worry that their vegetarian children are not getting proper nutrition. They should relax; vegetarian diets can be extremely nutritious, as long as they are well-planned.

For the overweight girl, however, vegetarianism can be a one-way ticket to obesity. While some vegetarians may lose weight by filling up on small amounts of bulky foods, others tend to eat excessive amounts of sugar, starch, and fat. A diet of pure granola is not very healthy and will certainly make you gain weight.

Don't despair, though. It's possible to lose weight on a vegetarian diet—you just have to put more care into planning your menu. A well-planned vegetarian diet can be just as varied and interesting as one that contains meat, particularly since most people don't take advantage of the different ways to prepare meat anyway. Just a glance through a vegetarian cookbook shows hundreds of recipes for soups, breads, cheese dishes, egg dishes, vegetables, salads, casseroles, soufflés, and desserts. Somewhere in there is tasty, nutritious, low-calorie food. (See Chapter 21 for some vegetarian recipes.)

The only problem is protein. While good protein can come from plants, no single plant protein contains all the *essential amino acids* necessary for growth. Amino acids, remember, are the building blocks of protein, and the essential amino acids are those that must be obtained from food because they cannot be manufactured by the body. Plant proteins can supply all the essential amino acids, but they must be mixed to do so. For example, beans can be mixed with cereal grains such as wheat, rice, or corn to make a complete protein. This "cereal-legume" mixture is the basic principle of "multi-mixes," which will eventually be used to feed undernourished countries. Unfortunately, "multi-mixes" have too many calories for the purposes of weight loss, and other sources of protein must be found.

Food groups and the amount needed by adolescents include:

Number of Servings (Daily)	Size of Serving	Equivalent Servings
1. Milk group—4 or more servings	1 cup lowfat milk	1 cup yogurt 1 oz. cheese ¼ cup cottage cheese 1 cup soy milk
2. Vegetable protein foods—2 or more servings	1 cup beans	4 tbsp. powdered soy milk 2 to 3 oz. meat analog 4 tbsp. peanut butter 1 oz. dry, textured vegetable protein 4 oz. soy curd
3. Bread and cereals—4 servings	1 slice of bread	½ cup cooked cereal 1 cup dry cereal ¾ cup rice ½ cup granola 2 graham crackers 5 saltines 8 Wheat Thins

Number of Servings (Daily)	Size of Serving	Equivalent Servings
4. Fruits or vegetables—4 to 5 servings	½ cup cooked vegetables 1 fruit 1 cup raw vegetable ½ cup juice	
5. Eggs—1 serving	1 egg	
6. Fat—1 serving	1 tablespoon	

Obviously, if a teen-ager wants to *lose* weight on a vegetarian diet, all these requirements cannot be met. In order to lose weight, I prefer eggs, nonfat milk, and cottage cheese as protein sources, rather than the higher-caloried vegetable protein foods and legumes. Maximum daily requirements should include: 1 quart of skim milk (or equivalent), 2 servings of eggs, and 1 multivitamin pill with iron. The sample menus that follow fulfill most of the minimum daily requirements of the dieting vegetarian. A simpler plan would be to (1) eliminate fat, whole milk, and refined sugar from any vegetarian diet and (2) cut bread and cereal to 3 servings per day; weight loss should not be a problem.

Menu 1

Breakfast 1 orange; 2 eggs; 1 slice whole wheat toast with 1 tsp. margarine *or* 1 serving of cereal with skim milk

Lunch Vegetable soup *or* tomato soup (use skim milk); peanut butter sandwich *or* cheese sandwich on rye *or* cottage cheese; fresh fruit; skim milk

Supper Meat substitutes: 3-egg omelet or sliced cheese or bean casserole; yellow vegetable; green salad with tomato; fresh fruit; skim milk

Menu 2

Breakfast Hot cereal with sliced banana *or* 2 tbsp. raisins

Lunch Tomato juice; egg salad sandwich; gelatin dessert

Supper Carrot casserole; cucumber and yogurt salad; ½ cantaloupe

Menu 3

Breakfast   1 orange; 2 eggs; 1 slice whole wheat bread

Lunch   Vegetable soup or tomato soup; cheese sandwich

Supper   Rice casserole; broiled tomatoes; Caesar salad

Menu 4

Breakfast   1 slice whole wheat toast; 3 tbsp. cottage cheese; ½ tsp. cinnamon (try broiling this combination)

Lunch   Low-calorie cranberry juice; cream cheese and olive sandwich on rye

Supper   Egg Foo Yung; fried rice; sliced oranges

Menu 5

Breakfast   ½ grapefruit; cold cereal; skim milk

Lunch   Scrambled eggs with cream cheese and chives; tossed salad with vinegar

Supper   Fruit salad; lowfat cottage cheese; rye cracker; skim milk

Anytime   Raw vegetable; nonfat milk

14

Staying on a Diet

"I'm on a diet. Two weeks have passed, and I don't know how much longer I can hang on. What can I do?"

Face facts. It takes a lot of time to lose weight. It is not a short-term problem, unless you have only a small amount to lose. Even then, losing more than ten pounds requires two weeks of dieting and an additional two weeks of maintenance.

Motivate Yourself

What are you dieting for? People who have a strong reason for dieting, a firm goal, usually do much better than people who are dieting "for the hell of it." For example, most girls will lose weight for their wedding. Their image of themselves walking down the aisle, slim and beautiful in a dazzling wedding gown, is enough to motivate them to resist any temptation.

In spite of women's liberation, more varied career choices, and generally higher self-esteem, I have found that the most popular reasons for teen-age girls to start dieting are boys and bathing suits. Other reasons include going to college, family celebrations, school plays, and school dances.

For your own self-confidence and peace of mind, I have tried to emphasize that you are dieting for *you*, not for other people. Unfortunately, that doesn't often give you enough motivation to get through the difficult times of a diet. There would be very few successful diets if every girl were shipped to her own desert island. In most cases, you just *have* to have a special goal.

Stop the Grab Reflex

Staying on a diet often becomes a matter of putting your conscious mind between you and your "grab reflex." Your grab reflex is what makes you reach for something you shouldn't eat and put it in your mouth before you think about it.

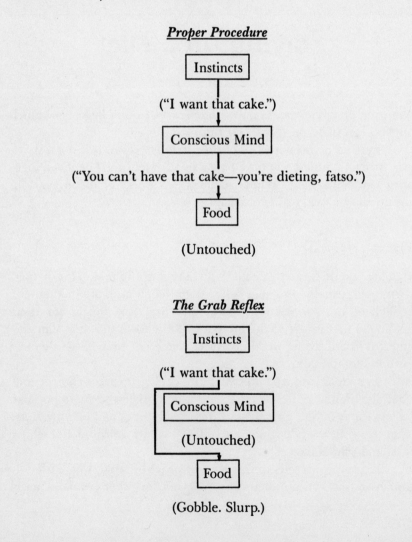

Proper Procedure

Instincts

("I want that cake.")

Conscious Mind

("You can't have that cake—you're dieting, fatso.")

Food

(Untouched)

The Grab Reflex

Instincts

("I want that cake.")

Conscious Mind

(Untouched)

Food

(Gobble. Slurp.)

Use your brain to give you time to consider whether or not you want that particular food. You might make the emotional choice and not the intellectual choice and take the food anyway, but at least you will have broken the reflex action.

Play Games

Dieters need gimmicks and games to stay on a diet, particularly after the first few weeks. Once you have settled into the monotony of losing two pounds a week, it's easy to get so frustrated by the rate of your weight loss that you eat out of boredom. The following games are meant to stall your compulsive eating:

1. *The Mirror Game.* Every time you feel like eating, look in the mirror first. If that doesn't stop you, take off a few clothes. If that doesn't stop you, strip down to nothing. Do you like what you see? No thigh bulge, no big butt ... then stop your diet! But, if you don't like what you see, keep dieting. If you must eat that piece of cake, eat it in front of the mirror and watch yourself swallow every bite.
2. *Word Games.* Remember the word games you used to play when you were a kid? One game that I played went, "If you step on a crack, you'll break your mother's back." You and I know that it's silly, but I never dared to walk on cracks.
3. *Making Promises.* Threatening to do something unpleasant if you don't live up to your promises to yourself is a common diet game. I have a friend who can only go on a successful diet if she swears on her sister's life. I know that sounds gruesome, but her diets always succeed.

Avoid Self-Pity

Sure, it's a bummer to diet. Sure, it's tough watching your friends pack in the food. But the more you dwell on these kinds of feelings, the less likely you are to stay on the diet. Everyday I tell my teen-age patients to be glad they have a disease over which they have *some control.* It's the old story—there is always somebody worse off than you.

Never Think, "It's All or Nothing at All"

Many people diet well for several weeks and then WHAM!—they eat a piece of cake. Then they say, "That's it—I've broken my diet. I've failed. Well, now I can eat what I want." And they proceed to binge wildly, eating every fattening thing in sight. And the next day they keep eating, reasoning, "I've destroyed my diet forever."

This all-or-nothing philosophy is the most common reason for diet failure. Don't let yourself fall into this way of thinking. In dieting there *can* be an in between, *IF* you are willing to go back on the diet after an interlude—whether that interlude is a bad night or a bad week. Just readjust your goals. You'll lose weight, but it might take longer than your original plan. That's okay! Time passes whether you diet or not. A few days more on a diet will be of no significance.

The real problem is how to get back "on the wagon" after you have stimulated your sweet tooth. Take a few days and eat only lean meat, lettuce with vinegar, and eggs. This will break up that carbohydrate cycle and get you back on your diet program.

Avoid Common Cop-Outs

Recognize an excuse. Be honest with yourself! Examples of excuses are:

> *Excuse:* I got hungry.
> *Positive Solution:* Eat nonfattening food.
>
> *Excuse:* I was meant to be fat; my mother was fat.
> *Positive Solution:* Pretend you are adopted.
>
> *Excuse:* I felt sick, so I ate.
> *Positive Solution:* Use medicine, not food, for curing illness.
>
> *Excuse:* I didn't have time to diet.
> *Positive Solution:* Make time. Cut your phone calls by 15 minutes.
>
> *Excuse:* I can't buy a diet lunch at school.
> *Positive Solution:* Bring lunch.
>
> *Excuse:* Dieting is boring.
> *Positive Solution:* Being thin is exciting.

Standing Up for Your Rights

When someone pushes food on you while you are dieting, staying on a diet becomes a matter of defending your right to be thin. This is called "being assertive" or "standing up for the rights of your body." That's the new emphasis in the more sophisticated weight-loss centers. Simply refuse to take the food that you don't need without being afraid of hurting someone's feelings.

Why do you allow food to be forced on you? Perhaps you think it is a way to be more popular. If you are overweight you think that you are less valuable than the average person and have to be more agreeable to be liked. And perhaps you really want the food and this is a good excuse for you.

You can assert yourself and be well-liked. People will respect you more. They might be surprised initially because that isn't your style. But styles change. No need to be angry or hostile—just sweet and firm. Have your own bill of rights that states, "I have the right to eat the food I want to eat without offering anyone any excuse for my acceptance or refusal."

15

Things That Interfere With Effective Dieting

In the course of a diet you will encounter many problems. Some of them are unimportant and disappear quickly. Others are persistent and often contribute to a decision to break the diet.

The Plateau

More diets have been ruined by plateaus than by anything I can think of. If every time you got on the scale, you got the kind of reward in weight loss that you thought you deserved, you would probably never stop dieting until you lost all your excess weight.

But when you have been dieting your head off for one or two weeks and you step on the scale and ... nothing ... zero ... goose egg, that's enough to make even the most determined dieter flip out.

Men lose weight in a logical straight-line fashion like this:

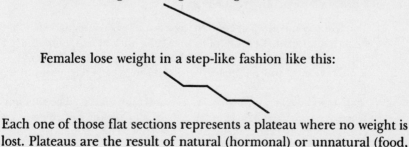

Females lose weight in a step-like fashion like this:

Each one of those flat sections represents a plateau where no weight is lost. Plateaus are the result of natural (hormonal) or unnatural (food, drugs) water retention. Water replaces areas where fat is lost, and until that water is excreted, your weight will hold stable.

Some of the times you tend to hold more water are:

1. The week before your period. Girls may have three effective weight-loss weeks per month. The fourth week you can forget. The body holds water as hormone levels become very high. Be content to stay the same weight that week.
2. After eating a salty meal.
3. While taking antibiotics for skin infections and other ailments.
4. While taking birth control pills.
5. After a Chinese dinner (because of MSG, a flavor enhancer).
6. After any meal high in carbohydrates, especially if you have been dieting. This is good for 2 to 3 pounds of water weight.

How can one avoid these periods of fluid retention? Many times you cannot. Just learn to understand them and not let them affect your morale. A few precautions might be helpful, though.

The day before you get weighed:

Decrease your salt intake.
Cut down on the carbohydrate in your diet (bread, potato, fruit).
Try lying down in a horizontal position 15 minutes after each meal or sometime during the day. This causes you to excrete more water.
Get weighed the first thing in the morning, after you have gone to the bathroom. That is the *only* time for a female to get weighed.

Physical Problems

Exhaustion

Many girls complain that they are exhausted when they diet and think that this is a natural part of dieting. If you are eating properly, you should *not* be tired on a weight-reducing diet. If you feel run-down, it might have to do with the following:

1. You lost too much water too fast, along with potassium and sodium. You should drink 4 ounces of orange juice with ¼ teaspoon of salt. If you feel better in the next several hours, your potassium level was low. Make sure you eat a banana or an orange each day until you feel peppier.
2. Your blood sugar dropped because you skipped meals. The solution is to take regular snacks at 10:30 A.M., 3:30 P.M., and bedtime—cheese, eggs, nonfat milk, or a piece of fruit. The solution is *not* to eat sugar.

3. You are slightly anemic. This means that you have too few red blood cells or too little iron in the red blood cells. Even slight anemia will give you symptoms of fatigue and listlessness. Get a red blood count immediately at a local laboratory. If found, anemia is readily treatable with vitamins and iron. If you are eating correctly and not having heavy periods, you shouldn't have this kind of problem.

Gas

Swallowing air, eating hard-to-digest foods, and food allergies are the main reasons for excess gas in dieting. Swallowing air is a nervous trait.

Many low-calorie vegetables like onions, cabbage, beans, and green peppers are hard to digest. Food allergies to milk, cottage cheese, and some hard cheeses also cause gas, either because of milk allergy or lactase deficiency. If this is a problem, you should take inactive charcoal or simethicone, both available in drug stores, to absorb gas.

Constipation

Constipation means difficult, infrequent bowel movements and hard, dry stools. Needless to say, it can be a very annoying problem in dieting. The bulk of the stool depends on the amount of cellulose—the indigestible part of the carbohydrate—in the diet. As carbohydrate is decreased, cellulose is decreased, and the stool gets smaller and dryer. Also, since a lot of water is lost on a diet, the intestinal tract is dry, and the smaller stools don't pass as well.

The way most laxatives work is either to lubricate or stimulate the bowel surface, add bulk to the stool, or a combination of the two.

Unprocessed bran is also excellent. It adds bulk to the stool by absorbing water and has a large, undigestible cellulose component. You can take three to four tablespoons per day (30 calories per tablespoon) mixed with orange juice or bouillon. This is plain bran, available in health food stores, not bran cereal, which is processed with flour and sugar.

Hunger

One of the biggest problems while dieting is how to keep from being hungry. Hunger seems to frighten most people, even though they have never experienced it for any length of time.

What exactly is hunger? True hunger is a physical sensation probably brought on by complete digestion of food. It is probably also associated with blood sugar and insulin levels. Hunger often expresses itself with stomach contractions. There are other body signals that people interpret as hunger, such as headaches, weakness, and fatigue.

It is normal to be hungry four to five hours after eating. At those times blood sugar levels are lower and the stomach is empty (emptying time is about four hours).

The problem with many overweight teens is that they respond to the sight, smell, and thought of food even after a full meal has been eaten. If you keep misinterpreting desire to eat as hunger, you must plot new hunger patterns.

Set times when you allow yourself to be hungry—8:00 A.M., 12:00 NOON, and 6:00 P.M.—and eat then. Tell yourself that anything you feel between those hours is simply not real hunger. Examine your reason for eating. Is it boredom (wanting to eat to pass the time)? Is it anxiety (using food as a tranquilizer)? Is it craving (longing for that special taste)?

Teen-agers diet best when they arrange their food intake in three moderate feedings (breakfast, lunch, and supper) and two small feedings (after school and at bedtime). This is enough to keep your blood sugar up and your stomach full. By small feedings I mean a glass of nonfat milk or a fruit, a glass of juice, a cracker, a piece of cheese, or a hard-boiled egg.

Real hunger is not selective; only the brain is selective. If you fill your stomach with things you *should* eat rather than things you *want* to eat, your body will be satisfied and your real hunger will disappear.

The desire for candy, cake, and bread as the only method of satisfying your appetite is a conscious choice and does not signal any special need. However, researchers now theorize that once a fat person eats a certain amount of carbohydrate, it triggers an intense craving that *is* chemical in origin.

Timing plays an important part in satisfaction of real hunger. The faster you eat, the more food goes into the stomach before it can register "full" and send the message to the brain. That's why you eat less when you eat slowly.

One way to do this is by cutting all food into small pieces. I observed this when my daughter had her braces tightened and wanted to eat a bagel. Her teeth hurt too much for her to bite into the bagel, so she cut it into ten little wedges. After she had finished five of them she said, "cutting it up into little pieces filled me up sooner. Now I can't eat the whole thing."

When you are eating fruits or vegetables, eat all the edible skins with the fruit; they also take time to chew. In one episode of the book *Pinocchio*, Pinocchio is starving and finds two pears. Being a rather finicky eater, he eats the white parts and leaves the skins. But he's still hungry. His cricket friend advises him to eat the skins. He eats them rather reluctantly, but is still hungry. Then the cricket suggests that he eat the rinds. Pinocchio is horrified, but his hunger is stronger than his horror, and he slowly chews them. At last he is filled up. That was very, very early behavior modification.

Another way to control hunger is to reduce the volume capacity of your stomach. First determine how much of something it takes to fill you up. Take a known quantity of food—a cup of cottage cheese, for example. Eat it slowly. When your stomach feels full, record the amount you have eaten. They try to cut back on that amount, gradually. For example, if you can eat a cup and a half of cottage cheese, cut back by a quarter cup per week for two weeks (one cup of cottage cheese is a reasonable amount to eat). By that time it should fill you up.

Food Allergies

Jody and the Oranges

Jody didn't really like oranges, but her parents had received a bushel of them in the mail, and her mother was pushing them that week. Jody thought they were too much trouble to eat—all those messy peels and sticky fingers. She wasn't wild for orange juice either, but she occasionally managed to drink a small amount. But now her mother went around repeating, "There will be no more food in this house until those oranges are finished." So Jody reluctantly began to eat them. They were the best oranges she had ever tasted, and besides, they were low-calorie. "Oranges that taste like this are worth the trouble," said Jody to herself, and she polished off six in the next two days. When she woke up on the third morning, the inside of her mouth was filled with canker sores. She could hardly talk.

Jack and the Hamburger Sauce

Jack loved hamburgers and was always looking for different ways to fix them. His mother came home one day with a new topping: a mixture of tomato sauce and garlic, flaked with bits of onion. Jack couldn't wait until he tried it. It tasted as good as it looked. About twenty minutes later his throat began to tighten and he had difficulty breathing. He felt as if he were having an attack of asthma, which he sometimes had around cats. But he hadn't seen a cat in weeks.

Cindy and the Egg Diet

Cindy decided to go on an egg diet. She wasn't crazy about eggs (in fact, it had always been a struggle to eat them), but she had seen a copy of a famous clinic's diet that called for eight eggs a day. She had two scrambled for breakfast, egg salad for lunch, two fried for supper, and hard-boiled eggs as a snack, plus two small salads. After two weeks on this diet, she lost eight pounds and couldn't even look at another egg. However, in a few weeks she had a craving for an omelet. As she broke the eggs and dropped them into a bowl, her eyes began to itch. By the time the eggs were scrambled, her eyes were so swollen that she could hardly see.

What do these stories have in common? All of them involve food allergies. Sometimes when you start a diet you eat or drink food that you would normally never touch, or else you eat larger-than-normal amounts of familiar foods and you develop an allergy.

Food allergies are strange. Sometimes you can eat a little bit of one food and nothing will happen, but if you eat too much, you'll have a reaction (example: Jody and the oranges). This is called an "All-or-Nothing" reaction. Sometimes you don't know which of the ingredients in a food is the one that caused your allergic reaction. Jack proved to be allergic to an additive in the new hamburger sauce, which was there to keep the sauce in a homogenized state. Sometimes you can eat a food one week and feel fine and the next week be violently allergic to it (example: Cindy and the eggs). Cindy became so allergic to the eggs that she didn't have to eat them—the smell of them set off her allergy. Sometimes it isn't one thing that sets off an allergy, but a combination of circumstances. A food allergy can be triggered by a cold or flu. A high pollen count or an insect bite (both potent allergens), added to minor hidden food allergy, will trigger a reaction.

Allergens can make you break out in those round, itchy bumps that we call hives; they can make you wheeze and have difficulty breathing; they can give you dry, scaly skin rashes; and they can cause your eyes, tongue, and throat to swell.

You might be having some problems and not even realize that they are from the food that you're eating. Have you ever broken out in hives (big, itchy, red bumps) from eating strawberries? Have your eyes begun to burn when you licked the spoon from the brownie mix? Chances are you are allergic to some food. Food allergies can do much more than make you sneeze or itch. They can make you tired, depressed, and restless. Recently I saw a patient in my office who said that she had been vaguely sick for a long time, and nobody knew what was the matter. Then someone discovered that she had a mold allergy. She wasn't eating moldy bread, but certain foods are produced by aging—cheese, wine, and certain cured meats like ham—and collect large amounts of mold.

In this country the most common food allergen is milk, our "most perfect food." This includes whole milk, dried milk, cheese, custard, cream, cream foods, yogurt, ice milk, and sherbet. Problems caused by milk include diarrhea (loose stools), constipation (hard stools), abdominal pain, asthma, headaches, tension, and fatigue. Also, milk will increase the mucus in the nose and in the back of the throat. Imagine giving milk to someone with a milk allergy and a bad cold: you'll just make that person more miserable.

Second to milk, chocolate and cola cause the most allergies. Both contain caffeine. Headache is the most common allergic symptom. If you've been getting headaches after drinking a cola or eating a chocolate bar, it's the caffeine that's bothering you. A friend of mine who was a peanut-butter freak had numerous severe headaches. Tests revealed that he was not only allergic to chocolate, but also to peanuts. When he gave up his favorite candy, he became headache-free.

Corn is another common allergen. It gives you strange symptoms. One set is called *allergic tension* and includes irritability, insomnia, oversensitivity, and restlessness. The other set is called *allergic fatigue* and includes sleepiness, vague aches and pains, and headaches. What makes this a serious problem is that corn is everywhere: in syrup, oil, cereal, prepared meats, canned fruits, jellies, jams, whole corn, cornstarch (used in thickening), and more.

Eggs. Some people just smell them and their eyes begin to itch. Eggs can also give hives and headaches and can cause your eyes, tongue, or throat to swell.

Other common food allergens include: tomatoes, which can cause eczema, hives, and mouth ulcers; wheat and small grains, which cause allergic tension and fatigue symptoms; peanuts; and citrus fruits, including oranges, lemons, limes, grapefruit, and tangerines, which all cause rashes and hives. Of all the spices, cinnamon is the most common allergen and causes hives and headaches. Some people develop allergies to hard-to-digest foods such as onions, cabbage, green peppers, radishes, cucumbers, and cantaloupe.

It is wise for all people who are allergic to common foods to wear a medical necklace or bracelet which states, "Dangerous Food Allergy: *(fill in food)*." It is also a good idea for them to carry a small, easily-dissolving antihistamine pill in their pocket or wallet. If they inadvertently eat something that's going to give them an allergic reaction, they can take an antihistamine as quickly as they realize they've eaten it.

Sabotage or Why Diets Can Fail

Problems in a Weight-Loss Diet

Sabotage is one of the most important problems that you will have to deal with when you are trying to lose weight. Look around you. Try to figure out where the most likely source of sabotage may be coming from. Is it ...

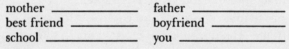

mother _____ father _____

best friend _____ boyfriend _____

school _____ you _____

A Likely Story

Jane and Roger had been going steady for two years. Jane wore Roger's insignia ring around her neck; Roger kept Jane's picture in his wallet. They were a popular twosome, and nobody would ever invite one to a party without inviting the other.

What made this romance the talk of the school was that Roger was extremely handsome—with a physique that wasn't to be believed—and Jane was fat. Not that she wasn't a nice girl; she was warm and intelligent and everyone liked her. But you couldn't call Jane plump; you couldn't call her round; you couldn't call her chubby; you had to call her fat. She always wore nice clothes, but they couldn't hide her round face, double chin, pudgy arms, and big hips.

There was a girl named Beth in the same class who would always mumble to the other girls, "I don't understand what he sees in her." Beth was really beautiful, with a body that elevated cheerleading to the level of high art. She wasn't a bad kid either, except when she got on the subject of Roger and Jane. Nobody held it against her, though. They understood that Beth liked Roger, but they knew she would never lure him away from Jane.

Roger's mother wasn't happy about the relationship either. She would say to him, "Aren't you a little young to be going steady?" which, of course, only made Roger reply, "I'm going to do what I want to whether you like it or not." Again, it was not that Roger's mother didn't like Jane. She certainly didn't object to Jane's weight—she was a little overweight herself and believed in big meals and in cleaning one's plate. Next to God and education, she thought, food was the most important thing in life. She even enjoyed having Jane over for supper because Jane didn't pick at her food like Roger's sisters.

Jane's mother and father were divorced. Her mother had walked out on the family when Jane was 12, and her father had remarried a short time later. Her stepmother was a tough, attractive woman who had worked all her life and still insisted on keeping her job, even though she had married comfortably and no longer needed to earn money. Jane was not terribly fond of her stepmother, and the feeling was mutual. In fact, Jane's appearance disgusted her stepmother. She talked it over several times with her husband and suggested sending her to a fat farm. But Jane's father laughed at the idea and said that as long as Jane was happy and well-adjusted, both of which she seemed to be, there was no reason to send her anywhere to lose weight. Jane's father was an old-fashioned guy whose own mother had been on the heavy side.

Junior year passed. Couples broke up and re-formed. Spring came, and Jane and Roger were still together and still happy. Beth, on the other hand, had gone through three boyfriends and had just about used up everybody in the junior class. She would walk by Roger and brush against his side—a whiff of perfume and a gentle rub—and say, "Hey, Rog, why don't you come down to cheerleading practice? You might learn a little something about sports." Roger just smiled. He understood Beth's hungry look, but never really took her seriously.

Toward the end of junior year, Jane began having trouble with her wisdom teeth. She went to a dentist who told her that they were severely impacted and would have to come out. He also told her that she would have to go into the hospital because it was too big a job to be done in a dentist's office. Jane had never been operated on before and was frightened of going into a hospital. But her dentist warned her that unless those teeth were removed, they would create a lot of problems, and she would be much sicker.

Jane went through surgery extremely well. Her teeth were extracted, but the anesthesia made her very sick, and when she got back to her room she couldn't stop throwing up. She was so sick to her stomach that the nurses had to give her a shot. They were afraid to let her go home.

Roger hovered around the hospital, extremely anxious. He cornered the oral surgeon and cried, "What have you done? Why is she so sick? She only got her teeth out." The surgeon explained that Jane had had a reaction to the anesthesia, and that because she had vomited so much, they were going to keep her in the hospital to give her some IV fluids. Roger was terribly worried. They had to shove him out of Jane's room when visiting hours were over.

The following day Jane went home still feeling sick to her stomach. She decided that she wouldn't eat much for the next few days because the sight and smell of food made her ill, and her swollen gums made chewing impossible. The weekend passed, and Jane forgot about eating. Friends dropped by with all kinds of goodies, but the sight of them made her sick. She thanked them politely and said, "As soon as I feel better, I'll taste all these nice things." Meanwhile she gave them to her brothers, sisters, father, and stepmother. Roger, of course, was around the whole weekend asking if she wanted or needed anything.

Monday morning Jane started to feel better. While she was dressing for school she noticed that her jeans were loose. When she went to lunch that day, she realized that her short illness had left her without much of an appetite. Besides, it still hurt to chew. She reasoned, "Why should I bother eating very much if I'm not hungry?" So she decided to have a small lunch. At supper she did the same thing.

After a week of reduced eating, Jane noticed—although nobody else did—a great difference in the way she looked. Her complexion was getting better; her cheeks were pinker; and it even seemed to her that her hair was looking a little thicker and shinier. Her nails were certainly doing much better—she had never been able to grow them beyond the nail bed, and now she actually had three that could be filed.

Jane decided to do something that nobody had ever been able to convince her to do: she would try to lose weight. She also decided not to tell anybody.

Weeks went by and Jane lost between one and two pounds a week. She lost weight throughout the summer, exercised regularly, and by the time she got back to school in the fall, she looked like all the other girls (except maybe a little better because everybody had been used to seeing her heavy). Jane and Roger were still going together, although there were periods during the summer when she felt he was hanging around too much. She really wanted the opportunity to get to know other boys. Finally, a lot of things that she had heard about being too young to go steady began to make sense to her. On her first day back at school she was approached by three or four male classmates who had known her for years, but had never paid attention to her. They all wanted to talk to her, to go out for a soda, and one even asked for a date. She was very flattered, but told them quite honestly that she was still going with Roger.

Things at home changed, too. As Jane lost weight, her father became very excited about buying her new clothes. He showed her off as if she were a brand-new possession or toy. She could go into any store and buy three or four sweaters or skirts. She had always hated to go shopping before because she didn't want to look in the mirror; now it was a treat. Jane's stepmother became rather irritable. Instead of being happy that Jane could finally get pretty clothes like the other girls, she appeared to be jealous. Jane told herself that she was imagining it.

Everybody in school was happy for Jane. Except Beth. Beth viewed every other girl as competition, but up until now the only thing she had held against Jane was Jane's relationship with Roger. But Beth had always had the other boys. Now she began to see her loyal slaves gravitate toward Jane. She got angrier and angrier.

One day Jane opened the door of her locker and saw a peculiar thing: a big box of chocolates. "How did this get here?" screamed Jane. Chocolates had been her favorite food, and she hadn't touched them all summer. They smelled marvelous. The locker was full of chocolate smells. Somebody's playing a terrible joke on me, she thought.

Jane quickly grabbed the box of chocolates and ran down the hall to the school office. "Miss Surpak," she said, "somebody just gave me a present. You know chocolates are terrible for my complexion, so here—why don't you take the box and share it with everybody in the office? Be sure to give some to the principal."

The secretaries were delighted, the way old school secretaries are when a student does something nice for them. "Imagine Jane giving us a box of candy!" they exclaimed.

The following day Jane went to her locker, and this time, instead of a box of chocolates, she found a big bag of potato chips. They had been opened a tiny bit at the top, and the odor of the chips saturated the entire locker. "This is ridiculous!" yelled Jane.

"It doesn't sound so terrible," said her friend Laura, later. "I wish somebody would put food in my locker." Laura weighed 90 pounds. Jane gave her the bag of potato chips.

How short people's memories are, thought Jane. They knew darn well that she had been a blimp a year before. Didn't they realize the kind of work and discipline it had taken to get thin? To stay thin?

The following day Jane was relieved to find nothing in her locker. She figured that whoever it was had given up. But on Monday afternoon she broke for third period and went to her locker early. She opened the door and again there was food—a 5-pound Hershey bar. She had never seen anything like it. She had seen little Hershey bars that were under 3 ounces, but never 5 pounds of chocolate! This was too much. Jane stormed up to the office. "I've got to talk to the principal," she said.

She waited half an hour for the principal to return from an appointment. When he arrived—a plump, long-winded gentleman—Jane explained the situation. "Somebody's trying to get me fat, and I don't know why. Who would do such a terrible thing?" she asked.

The principal nodded slowly. "You're right, Jane," he said. "It *is* a terrible thing. Besides, opening your locker is a dishonest thing to do. It's an invasion of your privacy, and we'll try to help you find out who's doing it. Meanwhile—um—can I have some of that Hershey bar?" Jane handed over her 5-pound Hershey bar, somewhat reluctantly, because by this time the temptation was getting to her. She wondered if just one square of chocolate would hurt her that much. She decided that it would.

The next day, the principal instructed a few of the hall monitors to watch Jane's locker carefully during periods. Jane was instructed to go about her usual business and to act as if nothing special were going on. The first period went by, and the monitor saw nothing. Second period was also uneventful. But 15 minutes into third period the monitor saw someone approach Jane's locker with a brown bag. The person opened the door, took a box of donuts out of the bag, shoved it into the locker, and left very quickly.

Jane went to see the principal during lunch period. She found him in his office, finishing off the box of donuts. "Want a donut?" he asked, and then stopped himself. "Ooops, sorry."

"Did you find out who was doing it?" asked Jane.

"We sure did. Betcha can't guess who it was."

"Beth?"

"No."

"My stepmother?"

"No."

"Who?"

The principal stopped chewing and looked at her. "Your boy-friend, Roger."

Roger! Popular, outgoing, devoted Roger! Why?

That afternoon a conference was arranged in the principal's office. A guidance counselor, Roger, and Jane were present. "I didn't think that I was doing such a terrible thing," said Roger. "As Jane got thinner and prettier, I really thought I was losing her. I couldn't stand that. I wanted her to be the good old fat Jane who was totally devoted to me and didn't look at anybody else. And nobody else looked at her."

Jane's first emotion was fury. Then she calmed down a little and suddenly felt very sad. "Roger," she said, "I'm just beginning to see myself as a real person. I think that we've gone together too long. I need my freedom. I need to grow, and you need to grow, too. We have been stifling each other. Maybe after I look around and make more friends and get to know more people, I'll find that you are still the person I will want to spend the most time with. But until that time, let's just be friends."

The meeting broke up. "There's really no disciplinary action to take against you, Roger," said the principal. "Just as long as you straighten out your act, fella. I'm sure this has taught you a very big lesson. No two people can entirely control each other. Human beings must have the freedom to move, to grow, and to expand socially and intellectually. You might not realize it now, but Jane's losing weight and asserting her independence is going to be just as good for you as it will be for her. Oh ... and where did you buy those donuts?"

This story is a blatant example of sabotage. Sabotage is any destructive act designed to stop progress in a certain direction. Jane was going in the direction of losing weight. Roger tried to stop her by placing tempting goodies in her locker.

One reason I told this improbable story was to point out that when a girl becomes thinner she has a new self-image. She feels much better about herself and is willing to take chances she would not have taken before. This could create problems with family and friends. Sometimes it is obvious sabotage, as in Jane's case; sometimes it is subtle. Often it is conscious; more often the saboteur does not realize what he/she is doing.

Consider a happily married, overweight woman who is busy raising her family. She has no desire to seek employment because home is both comfortable and protective. Then she finds she must go to work to help with family finances. While she is working, she loses weight and gains more confidence. Soon, she realizes that staying home was an escape and she really enjoys working. A supportive husband would encourage this independence, but an immature one would feel threatened. He won't force her to stop work directly, but he might try to make her gain weight again so she will lose her self-confidence and leave work. This is sabotage.

There are three types of saboteurs you should be aware of so you can protect yourself: the outside saboteur, the inside saboteur, and the worst saboteur.

The Outside Saboteur: Outside Your Family

Many girls tell me about boyfriends who start taking them out to dinner just as they are getting thin. I can remember a boyfriend I had in college. He loved to take me out to eat. In those days my favorite food was cherry pie. On every date we went to a different restaurant or diner so that I could sample their cherry pie. Of course I ate it with vanilla ice cream. My boyfriend was delighted to go along with this crazy behavior. I guess he felt that keeping me fat would keep me out of circulation.

Not all boys try to keep you fat because they are insecure. There are still occasionally boys who seem to enjoy plump girls. They say they want "something to hold onto," a good excuse for you to keep yourself 20 to 30 pounds overweight. There are several drawbacks to going with this type of boy. It's fine if *you* want to stay overweight or to run the risk of getting fatter. But if you want to lose weight, he may try to sabotage you. If he succeeds and then breaks up with you later, you may not find a lot of boys who you like and who share his taste.

Some friends will sabotage you to protect you from the change in personality that they imagine will occur when you lose weight. Friends know what to expect of you when you are heavy. You are probably pleasant and easy-going. They are afraid that when you get thin, you will become snobbish, arrogant, and vain.

Never underestimate the fact that being fat makes someone else look thinner. At one of my teen discussion groups the subject turned to dating. One girl said, "I always date enormous boys so I look petite beside them." There are a lot of girls who think this way about other girls. They love the feeling of being skinny beside someone who is much larger. It's really too bad that they have to get their kicks by comparing themselves to others less fortunate.

Learn how to handle outside saboteurs firmly, but gently. Never let on that you know what they're doing. Resist their offers of food with answers like "I'm not hungry now." At first, no one will notice you dieting. You will start to look better, but nobody will realize why. They'll think that you've done something to your hair. You might get compliments like "You have a very becoming new hairdo" or "Are you wearing some new kind of makeup? Your face looks so pretty." Only after you've lost 10 to 15 pounds will they begin to realize that you have been dieting. By that time you should have sufficient momentum to help you resist their efforts to fatten you up again.

The Inside Saboteur

The biggest problem for the teen-age dieter is the inside saboteur or the "household hypocrite." Teen-agers often find that adults are two-faced about dieting. Take the mother who (on the surface) wants her daughter to diet and then undermines her daughter's efforts.

Sarah was a very heavy teen-ager who wanted to lose weight before she went to college. With full family support—or so it seemed—she came to my office. She proved to be a model patient and lost 70 pounds or, as we say jokingly, half a person. She was well-informed, happy, and extremely proud of herself. But something strange happened to her family. As Sarah became thinner, they became angrier. They began acting as if her need for low-calorie food was a burden on them. Instead of being "good Sarah" who was successfully sticking to her diet, she became "bad Sarah" who was stubborn and fanatical.

They began to make little comments about her looks like "Your face is getting too thin" or "Your color is so bad you look positively yellow." Then came the gentle yet firm insistence that she eat. "Here, this won't hurt you, you're getting too thin" or "This isn't fattening." I would like to have reported that Sarah was strong enough to resist the efforts of her family to fatten her up, but, unfortunately, many former fatties retain the desire to eat the foods that made them fat. The combination of this desire and her family proved to be too tough an enemy for Sarah. She gained back her 70 pounds and was fat when she went to college.

Consider the process of family sabotage. It does not happen in the beginning of a diet. It occurs when the family gets bored and tired of putting out extra effort. There are three definite steps to sabotage, as illustrated by Sarah's story.

1. *Name-calling.* You are called stubborn or fanatical because you are determined to keep dieting.
2. *Undermining your new appearance.* "Your face looks thin" or "How did you get those circles under your eyes?"
3. *Insisting you return to eating.* "You're tired because you're not eating well" or "You really should not skip meals."

Is it surprising that most teen-agers who diet are furious with their families (particularly their mothers)?

Who is the inside saboteur?

1. The person who encourages you to lose weight and at the same time feeds you.
2. The person who wants you to cut down your calories, yet places all kinds of goodies in front of you.
3. The person who says, "Keep out of the kitchen," and then says, "I'm too tired to prepare special foods for *you.*"
4. The person who offers to send you for professional help, but, if you're not progressing as rapdily as he/she thinks you should, says, "I've spent enough money on you."
5. The person who doesn't know it all, but believes him/herself to be an authority on nutrition and diet.
6. The person who sees things in two ways—his/her way and the wrong way.

Home saboteurs are insidious. They bring cookies and candies into the house even though they know that's your weakness. They claim that they mustn't deprive the rest of the family, even though the rest of the family doesn't need a high-carbohydrate diet. They tell you that they are testing your willpower by putting goodies in front of you. They refuse to believe that sin is directly related to the amount of temptation. They will undermine you when you are doing well and become hysterical when you don't eat and hysterical when you do.

How can you handle them?

1. Learn to refuse them without antagonizing them; ignore them without being rude.
2. Filter out the useful things that they are saying.
3. Fight back your anger at the injustice of it all.
4. *Don't* eat out of anger, frustration, or hostility! Do not start or stop eating to spite anybody.

The Worst Saboteur

You. "Me?" You. "How?"

1. By not planning ahead what you are going to eat.
2. By not making sure there are low-calorie foods available at peak hunger times like after school or late in the morning.
3. By gulping down your food and believing that if you eat and run, you won't gain weight.
4. By listening to the phony advertising claims that promise pills to melt away fat, foods that combine chemically to help you lose weight faster, or exercising devices and bodysuits that will literally squeeze fat out of certain places.
5. By thinking that there is any better way to lose weight than simply decreasing caloric intake and increasing energy output.
6. By getting discouraged when you haven't lost as much weight as you think you should have.
7. By making excuses for overeating while you are on vacation or studying for a test.
8. By not looking in mirrors, trying on clothes, or facing the reality of your appearance.

I don't want you to go around suspecting that anybody who offers you a meal is trying to fatten you up. On the other hand, I don't want you to gobble down food you shouldn't be eating just to make other people happy or to relieve somebody else's anxiety. You must be the only person to determine your body size, so long as it is a reasonable and sensible size. Until you free yourself from other people and become an independent human being—at least emotionally independent—you will never get thin or most important, stay thin.

16

Tough Spots

During the course of any diet, you will run into many situations where you will wonder how you can possibly stay on a diet. During these times you must draw upon your knowledge, your ability to make appropriate choices, and your tact. You should:

> analyze the situation
> look for alternatives
> choose the one that will harm you the least

Many of these situations are such common diet hazards that I want to point them out to you in advance. I call them "Tough Spots," and if you learn to deal with them, it's half the battle.

After-School Appetite

"The school bus lets me out at 3:30 P.M., and no one is home. Mom gets home from work at 5:30 P.M. I am alone, and the only thing I want to do is eat. If there are cookies or potato chips around, I'll eat until I'm ready to burst. If Mom keeps fattening stuff out of the house, I just make myself sugar bread."

If you are dieting and these hours are tough to get through without eating, there are two possibilities: stay out of the house or busy yourself in the house.

1. *Stay out of the house.* This is the wisest choice if it is at all possible. Study in the library, get an after-school job, take up extracurricular activities that will keep you after school, and learn how to use public transportation.

2. *Keep busy at home.* If it is impossible to stay away from home (and dieting teen-agers always love to tell me something is impossible, meaning, "I don't want to take the time or effort to do it and I'd rather eat anyway), then you must try to regulate your behavior at home. Make sure that you have low-calorie foods available.

   Go for a jog; tackle an unpleasant task (such as cleaning your room); develop skills that occupy both hands (such as practicing the piano); whip up a lovely, low-calorie supper that the rest of the family will enjoy. You *can* work off some of your interest in food without actually overeating.

   Do seasonal things (such as making Christmas ornaments, planting vegetables, potting plants, shoveling snow, building an igloo). Do things to enrich yourself (like reading a good book—allow yourself one low-calorie snack to read with and then *don't move*). If all else fails, call a thin friend and visualize her figure, thinking "that could be me."

In our town after school, mothers line the driveways waiting to chauffeur their teen-age daughters home. You would be in better shape if you jogged home. If it's available, learn to use public transportation. It can free your mother and make you more mobile and less dependent. It also takes more time, so you will have less time to eat.

On-the-Job Temptations

"I just got a job in a pizza restaurant. I need the money so I can't afford to quit."

A lot of teen-agers end up working in places somehow connected with food preparation. Among my patients, I have two girls who work at a donut shop, three or four that work behind bakery counters at local food markets, two in pizza shops, one in an ice-cream store, a dozen waitresses, three cocktail waitresses, several countergirls in fast-food chains, and innumerable food checkers in food markets.

I don't know whether girls with weight problems seek out these kinds of jobs or if they are the only jobs available; but for whatever reason, working around food can be dangerous.

For those of you who work with sweets, the solution is simple—just eat *nothing*. There are no ifs, ands, or buts. *Nothing*. Work harder, faster, and more frantically than anybody else just to keep yourself busy. Even volunteer to help do something that isn't your job—make cupcakes, cut rolls, store candy—anything to keep you busy. If you work hard enough, you can reach a point where you are too physically exhausted to eat.

Ignore smells. Force yourself to forget them—it *can* be done. Smells by themselves mean nothing; they are interpreted in the head. Analyze what's in the smell that's getting to you, and convince yourself that it's *horrible*. Baked bread, for example, is not "heavenly": the yeast smells sour and the butter rancid. What's so good about that?

I tried this method with fried chicken. Every time I was on an important diet, my kids would buy fried chicken. There I was, sitting in the car with that marvelous smell. "This can't go on," I said. I decided not to throw away the leftover chicken and left it in the car in the heat. The next day I opened the door of the car and was greeted by the greasy, slightly rancid, thoroughly disgusting smell of what had been fried chicken. I would try to remember that smell when I didn't want to eat chicken—cold, greasy, rancid.

Sometimes you can turn working in a restaurant to your advantage. After all, you can often get a good free meal. Girls who work in Italian restaurants can eat an antipasto salad, the fillings for the grinders, or even a few meatballs and sauce. Girls who work in hamburger chains can eat meat without a roll, salad (if it's available), some sliced cheese, and diet soda. The better the restaurant, the better the vittles.

New-School Blues

"I just started a new school and I'm scared."

The new-school blues afflicts many teen-agers. Fathers and even mothers are often transferred to new jobs, and the biggest burden of adjustment falls on the teen-ager, who has been jolted out of her comfortable environment and plunged into the unknown. For the overweight teen-ager who is already self-conscious, this experience can make her retreat more than ever.

If you think everyone is watching you, it's usually true. Most kids are excited when there's a new person in school. Even the tightest cliques will, if they find the right person, open up for someone new.

The problem is often that your appearance determines whether or not you are the right person.

There are kids who will like you when they get to know you, who will turn out to be good friends, but they are not necessarily the kids who will enthusiastically welcome you. They are shy, thoughtful, and cautious—like you. They aren't unfriendly, they are just waiting.

But some girls do find an immediate friend in a new place— food! Alone and unhappy, they come home from school and eat. But food is not a friend, it is an enemy. While everybody waits, you should do something besides eat.

Get to know the adults in school. They are much more responsive to your immediate needs. I have found that school nurses are some of the best, most delightful, and sympathetic human beings. They will gladly put you on a weight-loss program or at least weigh you at regular intervals so that your appetite won't get out of hand at this crucial time. Find out if you can do something around the infirmary.

Get to know the librarian, and ask her if she can suggest some books for you to read or catalog. If you have a free period, you might be able to help check out books. This gives you a firsthand look at what's good to read instead of what's good to eat, and you'll also come into contact with a lot of people. Get to know your teachers, too. Even the most difficult ones can turn out to be understanding and helpful. You can offer to do extra projects to fill up your empty time.

If there is a school play, try out for it. If you can't act, school productions always need behind-the-scenes people. There is nothing like a school play to bring people close together, and if you are shy, the situation itself will push you into contact with others.

If your school has a newspaper, try to be a part of it. Again, you don't have to be a staff writer—take pictures, do layouts, or even sell ads.

Join any club or activity that you choose. If there are none in your school that interest you, and you see a need, create it. When I was growing up I went to four different schools from eighth through twelfth grade and never felt left out because I loved journalism and would always involve myself in the newspaper. I would make friends when people saw how involved and interested I was. Other kids tend to get scared off if they see you glumly hanging around and *looking* for friends. So make them interested in what you're doing.

Tornados A-Comin'

"I'm going to binge. Nothing can stop me. I'm going to eat that box of cookies."

Binge eating is one of the most stubbornly resistant phases of all dieting. It's like watching a tornado approach: you can see it coming, you try to get out of the way, and all of a sudden it's over, and there you are sitting in the ruins—empty potato chip bags, candy bar wrappers, and cookie and cake crumbs.

Psychiatrists say binge eating results from some serious psychological problem and is terribly self-destructive. I don't see it this way. Binge eating is "freedom at last," an escape from the chains of being careful. It's a desire to break the rules. It's like getting drunk, except you get drunk on food.

The only problem is that the next day you are faced with a few extra pounds of weight instead of a hangover. Sooner or later a person who loves to eat and is under constant restraint because of her weight, will binge.

The trick is to control the amount and the type of food you eat when going through one of these explosions. The problem with binges is that you binge on sugars and starches. By the time the binge is over, you have not only consumed too many calories, but you have had the taste of sweet freedom. It's hard to put somebody back in diet prison once this has happened.

I have a friend who found a solution. She binges every week, but she binges on lettuce. She eats two heads of lettuce. After that she is so physically full that any of the things she *really* wanted to eat are no longer appealing.

In my last book I had a "cheat list," which was designed for the inevitable binges. The rules of the cheat list are:

1. You must cheat consecutively.

2. You may skip no foods.

3. You may go backward on the list once you have eaten something on it.

For instance, to get to fruit you must eat your way through eight categories. If you go as far as fruit on the cheat list, you will hold your own or gain only slightly. Higher than fruit and up to ice milk, you will gain about one or two pounds per week. Higher than Item 16, you can gain up to five pounds per week. But remember, a cheat list is to be used only if you feel you *must* cheat; its purpose is not to encourage cheating, but to give you some kind of order to your binges. It organizes your cheating. Follow it from the top every time you cheat, starting with raw vegetables. Most of my patients get to about Item 4 or 5, then quit in disgust; they find it is too much trouble to work down to the food they crave. If they follow the list, there is a good chance they can successfully fight a sudden irrational desire to go off their diet.

THE CHEAT LIST

1. RAW VEGETABLES
2. COOKED VEGETABLES
3. EGGS
4. HARD CHEESE
5. SOFT CHEESE
6. FISH (CANNED, FROZEN, FRIED)
7. MEAT (PLAIN)
8. COLD CUTS
9. FRUIT
10. PLAIN POPCORN
11. IIIGH-FIBER BREAD
12. RICE
13. POTATOES
14. FRUIT JUICE
15. CRACKERS
16. ICE MILK or SHERBET
17. ICE CREAM
18. PEANUTS
19. POTATO CHIPS
20. FOODS SERVED CREAMED OR WITH GRAVY
21. NOODLES
22. COOKIES
23. CAKE
24. PIE

Party Girl

It's your sixteenth birthday and nobody remembered—or so you thought. Then you walk into the house, and everybody yells, "Surprise!" All your friends have made you the nicest party—pizza, soda, birthday cake.

There are certain times when you do what you must. Even though I feel you should assert your right to be independent of "food pushers," you can't *declare* you won't eat at your own surprise party.

Whatever you do, do it silently. Don't drink regular soda; drink water. Use the "rule of the halves" for this party. What is your ordinary pizza capacity? Mine is four pieces, so I'd eat two. Eat only half the piece of cake that is cut for you (slide the frosting off and just eat the cake).

Do a lot of talking! I have a friend who eats almost nothing, but she is so clever about it. She talks until after the appetizer has been served and then loads her plate with the main course. She takes a few bites of it and then gets involved in an intense conversation until it's time for coffee. Needless to say, she is very slender and nobody (except me) has noticed the game. I think she used to enjoy food, but she has probably forgotten.

Big Date Dinner

You are out on an extremely important date. The last thing you want to do is appear like you are dieting because some boys resent it, claiming that you are spoiling their fun. He takes you to a pizza parlor.

It is difficult to be cool about dieting when you are on a date. And, of course, cheap dates are the worst. It will take all your ingenuity to appear as if you aren't dieting.

Most grinder/sub/hogie/hero shops do have other dishes, such as antipasto. Antipasto is an Italian salad. So instead of a pizza or a grinder/sub/hogie/hero, order an antipasto. It has all the ingredients of a sandwich (lettuce, cheese, cold cuts, peppers), but no bread. It is very good and very filling.

If you feel you must take a grinder/sub/hogie/hero, take half the roll and hollow it out, leaving the crust. All the filling will fit into that hollowed-out half. No filling is great for dieting, but in order of desirability they are:

Roast beef or steak
Cold cuts (ham)
Tuna fish
Meatballs

Tell them to put no oil or mayonnaise (horrors) on the grinder/sub/ hogie/hero.

Girls often complain that they can't diet because their dates take them to *good* restaurants. That's the ideal place to watch your calories. Here are some suggestions on how to order:

> *Appetizer* (choice of)
> tomato juice; fresh fruit cup; bouillon or clear soup; oysters or clams; any marinated vegetables (mushrooms, artichokes, eggplant)
> *Salad* (any with oil and vinegar or diet dressing; cole slaw is okay)
> *Main Course*
> seafood and fish/plain; chicken/plain; tenderloin/broiled; roast beef; steak (any weight)/broiled; AVOID: Creamed ANYthing, curried ANYthing, and stews
> *Vegetables* (plain)
> *Potato or Rice* (baked or boiled with small pat of butter)
> *Bread* (forget it!)
> *Dessert*
> fresh fruit (if you did not have it for an appetizer); sherbet; ice cream

Order what you like and don't usually eat at home—not carbohydrates and starches. This is what makes eating-out fun.

Baby-Sitting

You are asked to baby-sit for a new family. You will have to eat supper there. You get there, and the mother proudly shows you her famous spaghetti that she has left for you and the kids.

Since many of you are at an age when you can baby-sit, this situation can come up often. Not every parent is generous enough to cook you her special spaghetti, but many of them will leave some peanut butter and jelly sandwiches for you to eat with the kids.

If supper is not included in the baby-sitting deal, there should be no problem. Take along a thermos of skim milk or a few cans of diet soda and a piece of fruit.

If supper is included, you have to declare your problem. Now before you mutter and mumble and storm, let me tell you how it looks from the parents' side. *Good* baby sitters are hard to find. THEY ARE JEWELS! And most people would be glad to help you out with your diet. It does not require any great preparation or expense; it only means having food available for you to prepare yourself. People who can afford regular baby sitters, particularly over the supper hour, can afford to have certain foods available.

A word of caution to those of you who take jobs as mother's helpers, particularly at the beach: some of the girls I've known worked like dogs for tiny amounts of money and were fed the most atrocious food, all for the privilege of a few hours on the hot sand.

When applying for a job as a mother's helper, tell your would-be employer that you will do a great job, and the only thing you require is a plentiful supply of low-calorie food. Most people will be glad to oblige. Good mother's helpers are harder to find than good baby sitters. Give your employer a copy of the diet you are following—don't assume she knows what to do. This gives her guidelines. And don't be afraid to cook your own meals.

Left Without Lunch Money

You didn't eat breakfast and ran out of the house with only a quarter. You are starving at lunch. An apple costs 30 cents, a cupcake 20 cents. You are too embarrassed to ask anyone for money.

School lunch seems to be a terrible problem for dieting teen-agers. Many girls prefer to skip them altogether. If you are on a diet, you should forget about your school cafeteria, but *don't forget lunch time*— bring your lunch!

I hear many reasons why kids don't bring their lunch: (1) I'm too tired to pack it; (2) There's nothing in the house to bring; and (3) There's no refrigerator in school.

If these are your excuses, you obviously don't want to diet. I know how difficult it is to function in the morning, but there is always the night before, and *that* is when lunch should be assembled and put in the refrigerator.

If there is no diet food in the house to pack, then there must not be any diet food in the house for supper—how can you diet at all? If you have diet food for supper, you can eat the same food for lunch— chicken, string beans, salad, hot dogs, sauerkraut, cold meat loaf, for example.

As for refrigeration, I think we Americans overdo it. When I was in Spain I saw many foods that we would normally refrigerate sitting out all day in stores and restaurants. I heard no reports of massive food poisoning.

While I don't suggest that foods with mayonnaise or anything creamed be left out in the hot sun, three or four hours without refrigeration in a school that is twenty degrees cooler than the outside shouldn't create a terrible problem. (Besides, you shouldn't be eating anything creamed or with mayonnaise.) Foods like cheese, cured meat (ham), raw vegetables, fruit, tuna salad made with celery and vinegar, canned meat or fish, pickles, and hard-boiled eggs don't need refrigeration.

I know you'll complain about eating them warm, but certain foods should be eaten at room temperature. Besides, you can buy little cans of ice now that keep them fairly cool. School lunchrooms are a good place to eat those "meals-in-a-bar" that have balanced protein, carbohydrates, and fat.

Lunch should be eaten sometime between 11:00 A.M. and 1:00 P.M. Many kids tell me that their school gives them *no* lunch hour, particularly on days when classes finish early in the afternoon. This is hard to believe, but if that is the case, you can have a piece of fruit between classes, and then eat something after school is over.

Back to our girl with 25 cents. If you are in this situation, borrow the extra nickel for a salad. Go to the office for a loan if you are too embarrassed to ask friends for money or to "cop" half a sandwich from someone (boys do it all the time). Or get a carton of milk instead of the cupcake.

Trials of Travel

You are going on a trip with your family for six weeks. They warn you that they have no plans to carry special foods for *you*.

Some families can be awfully thoughtless. They want you to be thin and then keep getting in your way. This is a blatant example of sabotage, and it will take all your wits to overcome it.

You must pack your own supplies. Buy food with some of the money you earned baby-sitting or from allowance or from Grandma for your birthday. Soldiers ate out of cans in the war and so can you. Get a good duffel bag and stock it with a one-week supply of goodies.

Your week's supply should include 7 assorted cans of fish, 1 jar of pickles, 14 small boxes of unsugared cereal (can be eaten without milk if no skim milk is available), 12 oranges, 6 grapefruit (for dessert and snacking), 12 cans of diet soda (if the family stops at a fast-food place that doesn't have diet soda, get a glass with ice), some dried beef (beef jerky), 8 packets of instant soup (tomato or vegetable, no noodle or rice), 2 boxes of melba toast, and 6 small cans of vegetables you don't mind eating cold (like string beans, mushrooms, zucchini in tomato sauce). Perhaps you won't need to use all of it.

Restock weekly as you run out. The first day out you can probably get a few things that are more perishable—eggs (which you can boil) and cold barbecued chicken (supermarkets sell parts of a chicken now).

When your family is eating beef stew, baked beans, and bologna sandwiches, dip into your supplies. When they are eating hamburgers and hot dogs, so can you. Learn to use good judgment. It takes planning, but at the end of your trip you'll be thinner and will probably have eaten better than anyone else.

College Food Fellowship

You arrive at college all excited and want to make a good impression. Your roommate is bone-thin. She offers you some chocolate chip cookies her mother made. Says they are the greatest.

Take the chocolate chip cookie and eat it s ... l ... o ... w ... l ... y. Tell her it is the best you've ever tasted. Don't eat dessert the rest of the day.

It is better to keep your eyes open and your mouth shut. You may find to your surprise that your skinny roommate diets like a madwoman and only pigs out with her mother's cookies. If so, she is perfect for you.

On the other hand, you might find she eats constantly, and the temptation of living with her is too much. One of my patients complained bitterly that the favorite pastime for all the girls in the dorm was eating junk food. Prepare yourself. Pack about 20 packages of plain popcorn for yourself before you go to school, so you can munch, too.

Assess the dangers of dorm living. Is there a place to buy food readily? Is there a refrigerator accessible? One problem in college is that diet food that's put in a common place like a refrigerator is often swiped. (Yes, in the best colleges this happens.) So while you refrigerate a bottle of diet drink, keep another unopened on hand. Also, keep several cans of tomato juice on hand—one in the refrigerator and the rest under your bed.

Buffet

You have been invited to the wedding of the year. You have never seen food like that. The buffet is huge and you are famished.
Choose well!

Buffets do not have to be trouble for a dieter. In fact, they are safer than lasagna parties. Let me give you an example of a modest buffet that was served as lunch at my hotel on a recent vacation. It included:

3-bean salad	hot peppers
carrot and raisin salad	ambrosia
green salad plus all the	fresh fruit
fixings	Jell-O with fruit
hot dog salad	yogurt
alfalfa sprouts	cottage cheese
chicken salad	cole slaw
baby shrimp	potato salad
chunk tuna	rice salad

I had a *feast*. I took green salad, hot peppers, shrimp, tuna, fresh fruit, and a tablespoon each of carrot salad and cole slaw. That was a fine diet lunch. I didn't ever miss the potato salad, rice salad, or ambrosia. I also could have made an acceptable diet lunch out of the following:

fruit with yogurt or cottage cheese
chicken salad and green salad
cottage cheese, tuna, and hot dog salad
tuna, fruit, and green salad

A rule of thumb about buffets is to take what is *plain*:

Plain meat, cheese, plain vegetables, plain potatoes, plain fruit
Take what has a protein base with mayonnaise—chicken salad, tuna salad, egg salad
Avoid hot dishes with sauce and dishes that are primarily starch (scalloped potatoes, macaroni, cheese, and noodle dishes)

Buffets can be fun and filling without being fattening.

Feeding an Illness

You have had an intestinal virus and have been throwing up. You feel better now, but the doctor tells you not to have salad or raw fruit for one week. The thought of meat nauseates you. Your mother is upset and wants you to eat because you look so terrible.

Mothers who scream about your weight one minute and force-feed you the next are all too common. The reason you look so terrible is that you have just had an intestinal virus; everyone looks terrible when they're *sick*. You have temporarily lost a lot of body fluids, along with potassium and sodium.

Treatment for a virus, particularly one that involves the stomach, requires:

resting your body
resting your intestinal tract
rehydration (drinking liquids)

Rest your intestinal tract. It's been sick. Would you walk on a broken leg immediately? Well, don't eat heavy food immediately. Have eggs, dry toast, artificially-sweetened applesauce, and baked chicken. Avoid milk or milk products or high-fat meats. In plain English, take it easy.

Drink lots of fluids that are easy to digest and low in calories. That does *not* mean orange juice, cola, or milk. Drink water, bouillon, or weak tea with orange (instead of lemon).

Soft Foods

Your braces were just tightened. Your teeth are killing you. Mother is having steak and mashed potatoes for supper, along with squash, which you detest. Dessert is ice cream.

The temptation in a situation like this is to eat mashed potatoes and ice cream, which won't hurt you for one meal. But if every time your braces get tightened or your teeth bother you, you eat that way, you will never lose weight. There are soft foods that are fine to eat. These include:

    baked potato (plain)
    cottage cheese
    Jell-O
    baked apple with artificial sweetener (baked quickly in a microwave)
    tuna salad with diet mayonnaise
    salmon salad with diet mayonnaise
    chili (see menu in Chapter 21)
    ripe fruits cut into small pieces (bananas, peaches, strawberries)
    - soup (vegetable or tomato)
    yogurt (plain) with one teaspoon of honey

All of these are perfectly acceptable low-calorie substitutes for full meals when you have a tooth or gum problem or even when you have a sore throat and feel you must eat.

Premenstrual Cravings

It's the week before your period. You are ready to eat the paint off the walls.

Premenstrual eating is often the ultimate feeding frenzy, and it can't be all psychological. There is definitely something hormonal about the need to put every carbohydrate that isn't nailed down into your mouth. A few tricks can lessen premenstrual cravings.

    Cut down on salt and carbohydrates for two to three days before your period. Eat meat and fish, eggs, salads (no carrots), cooked green vegetables (except peas). Drink water, nonfat milk, decaffeinated coffee, a diet *un*cola, and weak tea.

    This is the only time when I limit salt intake. Use grapefruit with artificial sugar sweeteners for sugar cravings. This will make those difficult days a little better for you. If your period is irregular, let your cravings signal when you should begin to do this.

    Vitamin B_6 (therapeutic level 5 milligrams and toxic level 2,000 milligrams) has been found to lessen premenstrual cravings in a dosage of 150 to 300 milligrams per day.

    If mood changes and swelling are severe, a mild diuretic or water pill several days before your period works quite well.

More Travel

You just persuaded your mother to let you go cross country with girls, but you are on a tight budget—$5.00 per day. How can you diet?

Dieting can be done on a budget.

> Don't eat out or, if you eat out, go to a cheap steak-and-salad place.
> Buy supplies a day at a time, and try to buy them in bigger towns
>   where there is not just one store. Look for competitive pricing.
> Buy small quantities so you won't be tempted to eat more.
> Take advantage of local produce or products (Maine lobster,
>   Maryland crab, Florida citrus, Texas beef).
> Learn to cook on Sterno.
> Use one piece of bread for a sandwich.
> When in doubt, eat eggs or unsugared cereal.

Turkey Time

Thanksgiving is your favorite holiday. Your mother cooks for weeks to
prepare and you know you'll never make it through.

I once read that the *average* Thanksgiving dinner adds up to 8,000
calories. That is 2½ pounds of fat, and God knows how many pounds
of water. Realizing what an eating holiday this is, a friend and I devised
a Thanksgiving dinner that is reasonable in calories.

> Turkey (white meat only)
> Gravy (get those new cups that skim the fat from the pan juices, then
>   take some *before* they are thickened with cornstarch)
> Cranberry Sauce (artificially-sweetened, whole berry)
> Stuffing (make stuffing with high-fiber bread, onion, celery, carrots,
>   eggs, water, seasoning; roll it into balls and bake it *outside* the
>   turkey; this saves 50 percent of the calories
> Potatoes (baked sweet with pineapple, pan roasted, or boiled with
>   parsley; normally, when you add sugar and marshmallows, the
>   calories are off the chart)
> Salad (use diet dressing)
> Vegetables (plain string beans with slivered almonds and turnips are
>   great diet food; just steam with salt and pepper)
> Dessert (we had the most problems with dessert, but this is what we
>   decided):
>   fresh fruit (tangerine, pomegranate, apple) or
>   nuts in a shell (work for them) or
>   pumpkin custard (take a can of pumpkin pie filling and combine
>   with evaporated *skim* milk and eggs; bake in custard cups;
>   this tastes marvelous and has half the calories of pumpkin pie)

HAPPY THANKSGIVING!

Beach Games

You are going to the beach with the gang. You don't want to carry *any* food with you. There's one food stand where everybody gets hot dogs.

Too bad you won't carry any food with you because it would be much cheaper and you would feel more satisfied. Since you won't, here is a plan that, while expensive, should not damage your diet too much.

> Hot dog or hamburger (or both), no bun
> French fries (small)
> Popsicle, fudge pop, or frozen custard in a cup

If you must nibble, choose cheese popcorn or thin straight pretzels.

Drink iced *water* or iced tea (artificially-sweetened). Don't waste your calories on sweetened beverages or beer.

If the food stand has fried clams, and you love them, get them; but omit the French-fried potatoes. Steamers without butter and corn-on-the-cob are good beach food if you are lucky enough to find them available. Remember, this is for beaching only, *not* everyday eating.

Sleepovers

You are sleeping over at someone's house and you refuse to ask your friend's mother to do anything special for you.

This time you *must* pack a few staples that have *no* definite odor: some cheese, hard-boiled eggs, celery, and carrots. Then survey the situation.

1. Are there foods you can eat with a clear conscience? Then dig in!
2. Are there foods that are "iffy" (casseroles, stew, spaghetti)? Use the "rule of thirds."
3. Are there just impossibilities (macaroni and cheese, garlic bread, and rice pudding)? Choose *one*, and eat half.

Unless you have encountered the first situation, you will still be hungry. You may do one of two things. Ignore it or retreat to the bathroom to replenish your stomach. Once safely tucked behind the closed door, you can eat your celery, carrots, eggs, and cheese with nary a telltale smell. If you were eating an orange, a garlic pickle, or sauerkraut, you would surely be discovered. You may feel somewhat silly sitting in the john with a mouthful of carrot sticks, but that is the price you must pay for not declaring your situation in the first place.

Night at the Movies

You are at the movies. Everybody is eating junk. You can't concentrate because of the crunching. Suddenly you find yourself at the candy counter.

Lucky you are that popcorn was invented and is sold in movies. Knowing you were going to the movies, I hope you skipped dessert at dinner so you can snack on a few cups of popcorn. If you don't like popcorn, look for one of those fat pretzels you can eat with mustard. If you crave something sweet, gum drops or licorice which, although they have sugar, take a long time to eat. Incidentally, low-calorie gum drops are ideal for movie munching (3 calories each). Buy five or six packages, and tuck one in your purse before going to the show.

17

Exercise

"I remember in gym I'd take something where I could get away with wearing a pair of jeans. I wanted to be on the swim team because I figured that it would be really good exercise. The only reason I didn't go on it was because there wasn't another girl there that was heavy. I didn't want to be in front of everyone in the competition. I would go for practices when it was just girls, but as soon as they put the two teams together, I didn't want to be there with a bathing suit on. I wasn't very active in phys ed at school. I would have loved to do everything."

A 17-year-old, 5'6", 170 lbs.

Anne, a teen-ager who lives on my street, always had a weight problem. She had been my patient, and she lost weight slowly—about half a pound per week on 950 calories daily. Unfortunately, she loved food, and in the face of her snail-like weight loss, she became more and more discouraged with each unsuccessful diet.

She came home from college one summer 25 pounds heavier than I had ever seen her. She started on a starvation diet and lost her usual half pound per week. But she was very nervous, and every time she felt edgy, she would eat. So instead of losing weight, she gained more.

Then she started thinking about alternatives to eating. She decided to jog because she had read that it was good for the nerves. I remember the first day she ran. In two minutes she was back home, exhausted. "I can't even get to the third house up the street," she wailed. But she kept it up—once around the block, twice around the block, one mile, two miles.

An amazing thing happened. As the summer passed, she literally began to melt away. She was losing weight normally for the first time on a 950-calorie diet. The exercise made the difference.

Most of my patients don't like to exercise and manage to lose weight just by dieting. They'll tolerate a few calisthenics for 15 to 20 minutes, but they resist anything as complicated as moving their bodies from one place to another. But there is a time in most diets when weight loss comes to a halt. "Your body is fighting harder to preserve that last bit of fat," I tell them, "so you must work harder to get it off. Eat less or exercise more." Usually they choose to eat less.

But when teens reach this difficult stage in dieting, I can't allow them to eat less: they are still growing, and their daily intake should not dip below 850 calories for any sustained period of time. So I tell them to exercise more. They respond:

"I'm too tired."

"I exercise enough in school."

"I have two jobs, so I'm always running around."

"I have a bad knee."

But I insist that they move. And their weight inevitably starts to drop again. These experiences, coupled with Anne's success, made me begin to realize that in this age group particularly, aerobic exericse is a *must* in effective weight loss!

Aerobic exercise is the type of exercise that steadily supplies enough oxygen to the exercising muscles for as long as the exercise is continued. Walking briskly or jogging for a period of at least 20 minutes, with your heart rate increasing at least 20 percent above its resting rate, is an excellent example of aerobic exericse. It not only helps weight loss, but increases heart fitness.

You can roll, twist, and stretch all you want, but nothing beats moving quickly. And it's not just a matter of calories burned; in the short run, they are not that significant. For instance, you must run 50 miles in 12 hours to lose one pound of fat. But only 50 minutes of daily swimming, jogging, or cycling over a year can result in a weight loss of 26 pounds, provided that food intake is not increased.

Don't look at exercise as a chore. Look at it as an important tool in weight loss, a positive discipline that will help you in anything you do, a means of keeping physically fit, a source of enjoyment, a way to tone up muscles and give you a better shape, and a cure for boredom and depression.

Also:

1. You expend more calories than someone of normal weight. So, for once, being overweight works *for* you.
2. Exercise raises your basal metabolic rate (BMR). You consume more oxygen, have more energy, and lose weight more easily.
3. There is evidence that regular physical activity reduces appetite by elevating body temperature and increasing breakdown products from muscle.
4. Exercise protects against loss of protein and muscle mass, causing you to use fat in preference to muscle.
5. There is a possibility that physical activity early in life restricts the total number of fat cells or will alter their size.

All of these things should be enough to send you running, not walking, to the nearest sporting-goods store for jogging sneakers and a sweat suit.

Why do you suppose overweight teen-agers have such a bad attitude toward exercise and movement?

I have already pointed out that certain body types are *not* energetic. The endomorph, or person of lateral build, resists exercise. Endomorphs have a naturally-low energy level that seems to have nothing to do with weight. Fat or thin, they're not energetic. That does not mean they can't get a lot accomplished; it just takes more effort.

Somewhere in the growing process, teen-age girls use up their energy. They seem to sleep more, wake up more fatigued, and tire more quickly than any other age group. Mothers are always taking them to the doctor to see if there's anything wrong with them. I always say they are "adjusting to their hormones."

The Home. Attitude about exercise is formed early, and the home plays an important part in its formation. Early exposure to recreational sports like tennis, sailing, and skiing often sets up a life-long pattern of exercise. Children tend to see parents as role models, so if parents are athletes, sports at this age are a natural outgrowth of a child's everyday living.

The School. This also plays an important role in the formation of exercise attitudes. Sometimes the school offers the only opportunity to learn sports correctly. The problem with our schools and our society is that they often place the overweight girl, who may not be naturally proficient in any sport, in a competitive situation where she is going to fail. This, along with her usual dislike of being seen in a gym outfit, makes her go to great lengths to avoid formal exercise.

When I was in school, gym was a nightmare. I was forced to wear an ugly blue gym suit and do everything with my "group." I remember my trials and tribulations on the gym floor: trying vainly to climb the rope and never being able to get off the floor; falling through the monkey bars; the list goes on. The worst humiliation was being picked for teams. The fat kids were always the last to be picked. We would stand huddled together, each hoping she would not be the last. In those days people assumed that if you were fat, you were poorly coordinated. I remember particularly wanting to play basketball— something about that sport appealed to me. There were 11 girls in my gym class, enough for two teams of five, with one girl left over. You can guess who that one girl was. Ever since then, I have felt sorry for those poor, chubby-legged, thick-waisted little girls in gym.

It was with that memory that I approached my local school system to find out what they do with the overweight, underexercised child. I found, to my surprise, that—at least in my town—things have changed. The overweight girl is no longer viewed as a freak. In fact, many of them are extremely able in areas like track, softball, gymnastics, swimming, and basketball. If their weight slows them down at all, they develop other qualities to make up for their lack of speed— endurance and strength, for example. Gym teachers tell me that overweight girls do beautifully in track, where they go at their own speed and are permitted to huff, puff, sweat, and not worry about how they look.

What pleases me even more is that schools are now interested in exercise as a means for each child to explore concepts of personal growth: sharing, respect for peers, and ability to face problems are emphasized at the primary level. Allowances are made for speed of learning, so nobody is left behind. And if a girl doesn't progress in a sport, she is encouraged to feel good about what she has already accomplished.

History of sports is also taught, along with a consideration of sports in our culture. Physical education has therefore become a mini social studies class, overlapping with such fields as philosophy and physics. Movement exploration and body management have replaced competition as the primary motivation in school activities. How can the body stretch, curl, twist, roll? Where is the body in relation to space?

There is a new understanding of girls in today's physical education programs. They are neither kept separate as delicate flowers not allowed to sweat, nor are they judged by male standards of performance. And all sports are available to girls, from dance to lacrosse to hockey. There are no sports that they are not permitted to try, although they seem to prefer movement sports to contact sports.

What are *your* favorite exercises?

Exercise	*Calories Burned/min.*
Talking on the phone	2
Talking in class	2 to 3
Talking in class and being caught by the teacher	4
Writing notes	2
Passing exams	2
Flunking exams	3 (you sweat more)
Riding a bike (not uphill and if parents permit)	6 to 8
Walking to a friend's house	4
Swimming	10
Gymnastics	10 to 20
Dancing	
Tap	8
Ballet	10
Disco	12
Cleaning room	
Voluntary	5
Under threat	3
Kissing	1 to 10 (depending on the date)

Any exercise is better than no exercise. You may be deprived of opportunities to exercise by well-meaning, but frightened, parents. Recently, a disco for teen-agers opened in our town. It is well-run and supervised, with no smoking or drinking allowed. But there are many mothers who are so uptight about it that they won't allow their daughters to go. Rather than seeing it as a positive activity where kids get some exercise, some mothers prefer to have their girls sitting in the house talking on the phone. They don't allow their girls to bike to the local shopping center or run around the reservoir. Yet they allow boys to do all these things.

If your family is somewhat overprotective, suggest to them that you be allowed to do these things in pairs or small groups. And once you have that freedom, don't abuse it, or you might find yourself once more sentenced to inactivity because of your parents' anxiety.

Exercise is the great equalizer—it makes you burn calories like everybody else. In order to lose weight like people who don't have as much of a weight problem, you simply have to move. It has to be *consistent* exercise, not normal everyday activity. Weight-loss exercise is done daily. Remember, disco dancing, roller skating, and biking are far better for your figure than staying home and letting your fingers do the walking.

18

When Do I Stop Dieting?

After they have been dieting for a period of time, many of my patients ask me, "Will I have to do this forever?" "Not unless you want to lose weight forever," I reply. A weight-loss diet should have a beginning and an end. Unfortunately, most girls go directly from weight loss to weight gain, so they often miss the end of the diet.

I usually try to encourage my patients to go down a few pounds below their goal, because they tend to gain weight when they stop a diet, *even if it's the best diet in the world*. When you stop dieting, you stop using fat for energy. The body then has the chance to pick up its 13-hour reserve sugar stores that were used up way back in the beginning of the diet.

Remember that weight loss you had the first two weeks? That was because you were using those immediate sugar stores. Each molecule of sugar you use held four molecules of water, and when you burned the sugar for energy, off came the water. At the end of any diet the sugar and water get replaced, and you gain back several pounds.

After the Diet

There's a diet after a diet. I hate to say that, but it's true. You have learned to lose weight. Now you must learn *weight maintenance*.

Maintaining weight is tougher than losing it. Maintaining is forever; losing has a beginning and an end. Maintaining is dull; losing can be exciting. When you are dieting, everyone is impressed with your weight loss, and you get constant feedback about your success. When you are maintaining, people forget how fat you were and the nonstop compliments, which you've learned to expect, stop. You are on your own.

First Month of Maintenance

When you reach your desired weight, you can eat anything you want except:

1. Foods made *primarily* with sugar (cakes and pies)
2. Foods made *primarily* with flour (bread, pasta)
3. Peanuts or potato chips
4. Whole milk
5. Fruit juice (except for 4 ounces daily)

Follow this plan for one month. While dieting, you weighed yourself every one or two weeks. Now you must weigh yourself *daily*, at the same time (early in the morning), without clothes, after you have urinated, and on the *same* scale. If from one day to the next, your weight increases more than two pounds, this is a significant gain (below two pounds could be fluid retention or premenstrual bloating).

If you gain more than two pounds, go on the following diet for one day:

Breakfast 2 oz. orange juice; 1 or 2 eggs (fried or boiled); 1 piece melba toast
Lunch 4 oz. lean meat or fish (broiled); 1 cup salad with 1 tablespoon diet dressing; 1 piece fresh fruit
Supper 5 oz. lean meat or fish; 1 cup salad with diet dressing; 1 cup cooked vegetables (no peas or corn); 1 piece fresh fruit
Snacks Raw vegetables, dill pickles, diet gelatin
Drinks Nonfat milk, tomato juice, diet soda, iced tea

Your weight will probably return to normal the next day.

It is important to record what you ate the day before you gained. You might find that there are certain combinations of foods that your body doesn't burn effectively. For instance, French dressing on your salad and a big steak might have caused that extra weight. In the future, when you eat a big steak, use diet dressing or plain vinegar.

A Diet After a Diet After a Diet

Usually, you can lose one or two pounds after a month on maintenance, if you follow it carefully. At that point, restrictions are eased slightly (although you must continue to weigh yourself daily forever).

For teen-agers. I allow one "forbidden food" daily. It must be part of a meal, not a snack. The rest of the day, use the Carefree Diet. Here are some possible foods: pizza, fried chicken, a milk shake, pancakes, spaghetti, fried clams, hot turkey sandwiches, waffles, or Whoppers or Big Macs. Remember, these are substitutes for your regular food, not additions to it. If you eat this way, your weight should stay the same.

Remember, no more than one carbohydrate—if it's cake, it's not cake *and* ice cream; if it's potato chips, it's not potato chips *and* pretzels. And it should be potato chips *instead* of a regular potato, and not potato chips as a snack. Pancakes can be your breakfast or lunch. *Again, remember*, you can't have it all. Some girls won't be able to have any. There are a few of you who will only be able to "cheat" once a *week* to maintain your weight. How often you can cheat depends on the results of your daily weighing.

Behavior Modification

Behavior modification works very well *after the weight-loss diet is over*. Weight-loss diets produce their own discipline, spelling out specific behavior changes during the time you are dieting. But once a diet is finished, how are you going to keep the weight off? Obviously, you can't go back and do the same thing that made you fat in the first place. Remember the three "R's": *record* keeping, *regimentation*, and *reasoning*.

Avoid Sugar and Flour

If you haven't already gotten the message, keep as far away as possible from refined sugar and only a shade closer to flour if you want to stay thin. Always remember what your critical level is and be aware that the level goes down at least one gram per year as you get older. For instance, if you are 15 years old and can eat 80 grams of carbohydrate without gaining weight, then when you are 20 you will only be able to eat 75 grams of carbohydrate to maintain the same weight.

Keep Exercising

Even though exercise is unpredictable for weight loss, it is spectacular for maintenance. Choose a sport or activity that will burn lots of calories, and devote at least 20 minutes per day to it. That will help you keep ahead of your sluggish metabolism and will keep it burning energy at a faster rate.

Be a Label Reader

What you see is often *not* what you get. Sugar is everywhere. Learn to read labels. If sugar is in any of the first four items on the list of ingredients, try to find a replacement for that food.

Don't Run Out of Low-Calorie Foods That Will Fill You Up

Everywhere you go, try to take something nonperishable and low-calorie in your purse. You might never need it, but it should be there.

Develop New Tastes

The more meat, fish, cheese, vegetables, fruits, and eggs you learn to enjoy, the less you will miss your previous high-calorie favorites.

Make Smart Choices

If you go to a buffet, look for food that you will spend a lot of time chewing. Avoid small, finely-chopped things that slide down your throat so fast you don't even know you've eaten them. Look for the lesser of evils. At a brunch in Boston, they served two desserts: a huge bowl filled high with a combination of whipped cream, coconut, marshmallow, mandarin oranges, and pineapple (I believe it's called "ambrosia") and some giant chocolate chip cookies. When you ladle the ambrosia onto your dish, you get more than 400 calories, and it goes down very quickly. One cookie is about 150 calories. If you have a mad urge to eat dessert, you'll do far more chewing, get far more satisfaction, and eat fewer calories if you take a chocolate chip cookie rather than the ambrosia.

Try to be aware of the ingredients in certain foods. If you don't know what's in something, assume it's fattening.

You are at a barbecue, and you have a choice of cole slaw or macaroni salad. You know you want to eat one of them. They both have mayonnaise. But macaroni has far more calories than cabbage, so take the cole slaw. Always choose the thing that started out with the least number of calories.

At a cookout, there is corn and potato salad. Both are starch, but the corn isn't mixed with mayonnaise. You might say "Why can't I have both?" That's how you got heavy in the first place. You could have half a corn and half an order of potato salad, but it's better to make a choice.

Get in Touch With Your Feelings About Food

Appetizers are something you eat before the main course to allow you to get in touch with your feelings of hunger and satisfaction. The premeals include a clear soup, marinated vegetables, tomato juice, melon or fresh fruit salad.

You might find you overeat if you rush food into your mouth without giving yourself a chance to realize you are full. Look at some of the overweight people eating so rapidly that they don't pay any attention to what goes into their mouths; or else, they become so engrossed in conversation that they forget they are eating. If you are one of those fast, grabby eaters, you may *cut* down by *slowing* down. Pause between each forkful; visit a while before going for seconds; the food will still be there (unfortunately). You may realize that you don't want anymore after all.

Make Calories Count

I have always tried to eat food that gives me the most mileage. If I sit down for lunch and am extremely hungry, I order a chef's salad; you get so much food nutrition for so few calories. That's the gripe I have with fruit juice. You get all the calories, but none of the chewing, so you feel you haven't eaten anything. I would rather you eat an apple than drink 3 to 4 ounces of apple juice. That's probably one of the reasons why I don't like canned fruit either; too many calories slide down too fast.

In most of my diets, I allow unlimited raw vegetables, and yet I restrict cooked vegetables. Why? It is almost impossible to gain weight on raw vegetables because they are so bulky and fill you up quickly. If you cook the same vegetables, you take out the fiber and the water—so you can eat much more of them without filling up as much.

I would rather eat 58 small pretzel sticks than 3 vanilla wafers or 1 cookie. I suppose I'd like the cookie more, but I'd get to chew the pretzels much more.

Baked potato snacks have a lot of staying power. If you eat the skins, they are quite filling and require lots of time to chew.

Dilute and Substitute

Whenever you can get the same taste for fewer calories, do it.

Diet margarine for regular margarine
Diet gum for regular gum
Skim milk for whole milk
Diet mayonnaise for regular mayonnaise
Diet salad dressing for regular salad dressing
Diet soda for regular soda

Some of the recipes in the recipe section (see Chapter 21) give you the same taste you want without extra carbohydrates and fat. If you are cooking, remember to use one third less sugar; most recipes that call for sugar are too sweet anyway.

Fructose is sweeter than sugar, so if you use fructose in the recipe, you can probably use one half the amount of sugar that is called for.

Don't Fall for Food Myths

There are many myths about food and dieting that we take as gospel, and often we allow them to determine our eating habits. People like to invest some foods with a certain mystique, and that's fine, as long as these myths don't interfere with your diet or nutrition.

True or False

1. Onions, oysters, and olives make you sexy.
   False. For girls, being sexy is in the head, not in the food.
2. Butter has more calories than margarine.
   False. Butter and margarine both have 90 calories per tablespoon. Butter is a saturated fat and margarine is unsaturated.
3. Milk is a perfect food.
   False. Whole milk is usually fattening. Milk allergies and milk intolerances are common in teen-agers. Milk does not have iron, unless it's fortified. Milk has probably caused more stomach upsets than it has cured.
4. Fish is brain food.
   False. Fish is a high-protein, low-fat food. Its value in today's world lies in the fact that it is lower in calories than meat, but still very nutritious. However, the more a fish resembles meat (like swordfish

and salmon), the more fat it contains, and the closer the calories are
to beef. If you like fish, eat it; if you don't, don't force yourself. You
won't become a halfwit.

5. Orange juice is good for a cold.
   False. I find this myth very irritating. If you have a cold, there is little
   you can do to shorten its duration. If you are trying to lose weight,
   one or two vitamin C pills are just as effective.

6. Eggs are bad for you.
   False. It's the old cholesterol argument. You, as a teen-age female,
   should learn to enjoy eggs and eat them as much as possible. They
   are a low-calorie, high-protein, inexpensive way to diet. Incidentally,
   brown and white eggs supply the same nutritional value.

7. Spinach makes you strong.
   False. Since spinach seems to be the most unpopular vegetable among
   teen-agers, you probably don't eat a lot of it. Popeye the Sailorman
   notwithstanding, it has no muscle-producing qualities, but it is rich in
   vitamin A and low in calories.

8. Toasted bread has less calories than untoasted.
   False. Unless you toast it very dark—like burn it black.

9. You can eat all the fruit you want on a diet.
   False. If you eat all the fruit you want, chances are you won't lose
   weight, and it is quite possible to gain weight if you eat enough of it.
   Fruit is a sugar—a natural sugar, but still a sugar.

10. Food eaten before you go to bed is more likely to make you gain
    weight.
    False. If you eat fattening food, it will make you gain weight anytime.
    If you eat a supper high in protein and low in carbohydrates, it
    doesn't seem to matter when you eat. New studies indicate, however,
    that carbohydrate foods eaten earlier in the day are more likely to be
    burned off.

Tell Yourself the Food Will Be There Tomorrow

Once I was sitting at a party with a man who was eating very little, very
slowly. The food at the party happened to be spectacular, and I was
wolfing it down. I said to him, "What's the matter, are you sick or
something?" He smiled and said, "There will always be food tomorrow
that will be just as good, and if I don't overstuff myself today, I can eat
all I want then."

Don't Think Thin

That's right. You should "think thin" on the way down, but once you
are there, "think fat." You are a fat person in a thin body. If you start

thinking you're naturally a thin person, you will start eating everything. If you start eating everything, you won't be thin.

Learn to Communicate

What does communication have to do with weight maintenance? It's so easy to eat in silence. Keep the lines of communication open between you and your family. Don't retreat from human contact or sulk when you think you have been wronged. Many times feelings of anger, frustration, and disappointment lead back to overeating. If you can express your feelings in words, you won't have to express them by eating.

The Scale and You

From now on, you must develop a new relationship with your scale. A good scale should be as important to you as a new stereo, so save up your money and try to buy one with balances (like in the doctor's office).

Regular bathroom scales are spring scales, and at best they only approximate your weight. They can be affected by jiggling up and down, humidity, or a full moon. Since you will be looking for small weight fluctuations (two to three pounds), it would be better to have an accurate scale. And please remember to weigh yourself at the same time every day in the morning. A female can literally starve all day and still weigh two pounds more at night.

Coping With Your New Body

One of my patients told me that she likes herself more as a person when she's fat than when she's thin. "When I get thin," she explained, "I get too cocky, too seductive, too sure of myself. I have a great feeling of power. I feel I can seduce anybody. I even send out sexual signals to guys who don't appeal to me. As far as girls are concerned, I become a real cat. I organize little cliques and exclude girls who look the way I used to look. I criticize girls if their figures aren't good. My budget gets shot, too; I want to buy everything that I look at. It's like a disease. I always looked so terrible in clothes, and now everything I try on looks great. I used to think about other things, but now it's always *me*."

She really said it all. I'm sure you will recognize a few of these traits in *the thin you*. And to a certain extent, you have to guard against them. Now, remember, I said to a certain extent. It is necessary for you to keep a moderate and healthy degree of self-love to preserve your new figure.

After the glow of thinning wears off and you've settled down to a "new" existence, you'll realize that although you feel better and look better, you are still the same person. But all of a sudden, you will start getting a lot more attention from the opposite sex. Girls who would have been happy with one boyfriend will now have as many as possible. It is amazing what just being thinner, without being better, does to a girl's popularity. It does go to your head and can make you cocky.

It can also be scary. You will constantly be wrestling with questions like, "How far do I go?" "How soon is it okay to have sex?" "Should I start taking the pill?"

Girls who have always been thin have made these decisions long ago because they have had to grow up with these temptations. It's easy to be pure if you hate the guys you're dating and you're embarrassed about your shape.

Your sexuality is a very potent tool. Use it wisely. Understand it. Don't let it overwhelm you. And don't use it to hurt people just because you were once hurt.

19

Calories

Most calorie charts strike me as inadequate aids for dieting. They employ inconsistent measurements—1 cup here, ½ cup there, 3 ounces, 6 ounces, ecetera.

The only time when calorie-counting is necessary is when you're on a diet and not losing weight. Then it might help to examine your total caloric intake and determine which foods are pushing you over your limit. That's why I'm going to include a small calorie chart in the book, which I hope will be of some value to you.

Why haven't I included calories in my diets or in most of the recipe section? I think it's more important to understand calorie *ranges* than exact numbers.

For instance, the diet for inactive teen-agers contains between 850 and 950 calories; for active teen-agers, between 1,300 and 1,400 calories. The crash diets are generally under 1,000 calories. None of the recipes in this book, if substituted for plain meat, vegetables, or salad, would jeopardize your diet. The "fattening" ingredients have been kept to a minimum.

I would prefer that you come away from this book with an understanding of the content of food (proteins, carbohydrates, and fat) and *portion control* (knowing the difference between a pound and four ounces of steak). You should recognize which foods are more likely to make you fat. This way you'll be able to monitor your eating habits for life and not just whenever you feel like taking an exact calorie count of a meal.

Modified Calorie Chart

Food Item	Quantity Per Serving	Calories
	Beverages (except milk)	
Alcoholic		
Beer	1 glass	144
Light beer	1 glass	80
1 oz. liquor	1 jigger	80
Wine, dry	1 wineglass	96
Wine, sweet	1 wineglass	184
Carbonated		
Coca-Cola	1 glass	104
Ginger ale	1 glass	80
Pepsi-Cola	1 glass	106
Coffee, clear, no sugar	1 cup	5
Tea, clear, no sugar	1 cup	2
Cider	1 glass	115
	Bread	
White	1 slice	62
Whole wheat	1 slice	56
Rye	1 slice	56
Zwieback	1 piece	31
Melba toast	1 piece	15
Biscuit	1	129
Bun, cinnamon	1	158
Doughnut		
Raised	1	124
Sugar and icing	1	151
Jelly	1	226
Muffin, white	1	118
Pancake	1	104
Waffle	1	209
French toast	1	183
	Cereal	
All-Bran	1 cup	190
Corn Flakes	1 cup	95
Grape Nuts	1 cup	440
Puffed Rice	1 cup	51
Oatmeal (cooked)	1 cup	131

*Unless otherwise specified, 1 glass = 8 oz., 1 cup = 8 oz.

Food Item	Quantity Per Serving	Calories
Fats		
Butter, dairy, salted	1 tsp.	36
Oleomargarine	1 tsp.	36
Oil	1 tsp	45
Mayonnaise	1 tbsp.	101
Blue cheese dressing	1 tbsp.	71
French dressing	1 tbsp.	57
Italian dressing	1 tbsp.	77
Yogurt		
Skimmed	1 cup	122
Whole	1 cup	155
Cream		
Coffee or table	1 tbsp.	32
Whipped cream	1 cup	420
Cheese		
Cottage, creamed	1 cup	239
Cottage, low-fat, not creamed	1 cup	125
Sour cream	1 cup	454
Cheddar	1 ounce	112
Cream	1 ounce	105
Parmesan	1 ounce	110
Swiss	1 ounce	100
American	1 ounce	107
Ice cream	1 scoop	128
Ice cream soda, vanilla	1 regular	261
Milk shake, chocolate	1 regular (12 oz.)	504
Milk		
Buttermilk	1 glass*	92
Chocolate	1 glass	205
Skimmed	1 glass	81
Whole	1 glass	161
Dessert		
Pie		
Apple	1 serving†	410
Pumpkin	1 serving	317
Pecan	1 serving	668
Cake, no icing		
Angel Food	1 serving‡	75
Chocolate	1 serving	234
Yellow	1 serving	233

*1 glass = 8 oz.
†Pie serving = ⅙ of a 9″ pie
‡Cake serving = ⅟₁₆ of a 9″ cake

Food Item	Quantity Per Serving	Calories
Dessert (Cont.)		
Pudding		
Chocolate	1 cup	438
Vanilla	1 cup	304
Diet gelatin	1 cup	20
Jell-O, plain	1 cup	160

	Fruit (raw)	
Apple	1	133
Banana	1	127
Apricot	1	21
Pear	1	122
Orange	1	73
Tangerine	1	35
Peach	1	38
Plum	1	33
Avocado	1	334
Cantaloupe	1 whole	120
Grapefruit	1 whole	80
Honeydew	1 whole	240
Tomato	1 med.	33
Dates	1	27
Figs	1	40
Strawberries	1 cup	56
Blackberries	1 cup	84
Blueberries	1 cup	87
Cherries	1 cup	116
Cranberries	1 cup	46

	Poultry	
Eggs	1	78
Chicken		
Roasted	1 serving	220
Broiled	1 whole	668
Breast	1 breast half	160
Stewed	1 serving	216
Turkey	1 serving	235
Duck	1 serving	323

Food Item	Quantity Per Serving	Calories
	*Fish**	
Crab	1 serving	93
Flounder or sole	1 serving	68
Lobster	1 serving	91
Salmon	1 serving	207
Shrimp	1 serving	91
Tuna, in oil	1 serving (small)	288
Tuna, in water	1 serving (small)	127
Oysters	1 serving	66
Sardines	1 serving	311
Scallops	1 serving	112
	Meat	
Chop		
Pork	1	357
Lamb	1	207
Roasts		
Beef, rib	1 serving	302
Beef, round	1 serving	254
Beef, corned	1 serving	240
Ham	1 serving	348
Lamb	1 serving	242
Frankfurter	1	124
Bologna	1 slice, 1 oz.	66
Salami	1 slice, 1 oz.	130
Liverwurst	1 slice, 1 oz.	79
	Vegetables	
Asparagus	1 cup	30
Beans		
Green	1 cup	30
Lima	1 cup	190
Mung, sprouted	1 cup	35
Baked beans	1 cup	376
Beets	1 cup	55
Broccoli	1 cup	40
Brussels sprouts	1 cup	50
Cabbage, raw	1 cup	24
Cabbage, cooked	1 cup	35

*One serving of fish or meat = approximately 3½ ounces unless otherwise indicated.

Food Item	Quantity Per Serving	Calories
Vegetables (Cont.)		
Carrots, raw	1	20
Carrots, cooked	1 cup	45
Celery	1 stalk	8
Corn on the cob	1 ear	96
Corn, canned	1 cup	140
Cucumber	1	14
Lettuce, iceberg	1 head	60
Mushrooms, canned	1 cup	40
Onions, raw	1	40
Onions, cooked	1 cup	60
Peas	1 cup	106
Peppers, green	1	15
Potatoes	1	140
French-fried	1 stick	15
Radishes	1	1.3
Spinach	1 cup	40
Tomatoes, raw	1	33
Tomatoes, cooked	1 cup	50
Sauerkraut	1 cup	27
Chocolate syrup	1 tbsp.	49
Popcorn	1 cup	54
Potato chips, etc.	1 oz.	140–170
Nuts		
Peanuts	1 oz.	283
Cashews	1 oz.	280
Mixed nuts	1 oz.	188

20

The Overweight Teen-Ager
Who Likes to Cook

Food, Food Everywhere—But Not a Bite to Eat

I'm not putting a recipe chapter in this book only because you are girls and girls should know something about cooking. I think girls should know karate, auto mechanics, *and* cooking.

Knowledge of cooking can be extremely important if you have a weight problem because:

1. It helps you become more self-reliant about preparing your own food.
2. It gives you an idea of what goes into foods, so you can order correctly at restaurants.
3. It adds variety to low-calorie meal planning. Chicken is chicken is chicken, but a few different spices and it's Mexican, Italian, or Chinese.

Learn to enjoy cooking because it is creative and fun, not something you must do because it's your role. It can be a great way to release tension—as good as needlepoint or crossword puzzles—and it is something that can give other people enjoyment.

My daughter just came home from her home economics class, and I asked her what they were cooking up these days. She told me they were making granola bars, applesauce, muffins, and cookies. Except for the granola bars, times haven't changed much. What do all these foods have in common? You guessed it, lots of sugar. Is it any wonder that the teen-ager who starts cooking for her family knows only about carbohydrate cookery?

Many overweight children enjoy food preparation. They have a talent for cooking, usually because they appreciate food. Some mothers frustrate their daughters' attempts at cooking because kids sometimes make a mess. Occasionally these mothers relent and allow their daughters to bake desserts for the family. While I don't advocate heavy cooking when dieting, I do think that no talent should be wasted. Instead of teens complaining how dull and uninteresting lower-calorie foods are, it might make more sense to allow them to cook some of them by themselves.

This will be a section of recipes and simple hints to spark up meals. I'm not going to include calorie counts because most of the recipes won't damage any diet when used occasionally. I have cut the higher-calorie ingredients down to a minimum, just enough to preserve the flavor.

It is the purpose of this section to stimulate an interest in *general* cooking as opposed to *dessert* cooking. Also I hope that it will teach girls some nutritional lessons. Remember, I'm a plain-food advocate when it comes to dieting. Broil. Bake. Steam. Keep it simple, keep it plain. But if you want to spark up diet meals, I will include recipes that will taste good without wrecking your weight-loss program.

Anyone who can follow a recipe can cook, and anyone who can follow a good recipe can be a good cook. It is more difficult and requires more imagination to be a good cook when you are on a diet and have to eliminate certain foods entirely. But the teen-age dieter who enjoys cooking can begin by following these recipes and suggestions for preparing some basic daily foods. After a bit of experience, learn to vary them a little to suit your own taste.

There are certain things that you ought to have in a kitchen if you are going to attempt serious cooking. Besides regular cooking tools, check for these important items:

1. *Teflon-coated pans*, so you can keep fat for frying down to a minimum.
2. *Food-measuring equipment.* A good cook follows a recipe exactly until she is experienced and knows enough to be able to improvise.
3. *Food scale.*
4. *Sharp knives.* These are important. There's nothing more frustrating than trying to hack away at vegetables or meat with a dull knife. (I'll never understrand why a father will give a penknife to his son and get uptight when his daughter uses a kitchen knife.)
5. *Vegetable brush* for scrubbing. Many people advocate scrubbing veggies, instead of peeling them, since so many vitamins reside in the skins.

6. *Assortment of herbs.* These add different flavors to your food. Get acquainted with garlic, basil, oregano, thyme, rosemary. Smell them. Rub them between your fingers; see if you can identify them in different foods.

7. *A good recipe book.* I object to recipe books that are especially geared for children, just as I object to classic books that are watered down (or "abridged") so children can read them more easily. What you need is a recipe book that defines basic cooking procedures and gives you some instruction. Most important, perhaps, it should have a little explanation about individual dishes and their ingredients. A little bit of food history is fun, also.

8. *Plenty of lemons.* Lemons are a great natural taste enhancer and can be used on many foods.

9. *A small steamer.* This can be one of those fold-up jobs that can be purchased at any kitchen shop or hardware store for a few dollars. You'll discover a whole new world of texture and taste when you steam vegetables instead of boiling them.

10. *A calorie chart*—just for comparison's sake. These can be purchased in most drugstores that carry paperbacks or in bookstores. After you become familiar with the relative calorie content of different foods, it will be easier for you to make changes in recipes.

If you are really fortunate and have a progressive parent, you may have a food processor in the kitchen. This is a marvelous tool. It can slice, chop, purée, shred, and shoestring. It can cut kitchen time in half (also your finger, if you are not careful). Make sure you know how to use it *before* you attempt to slice something.

Snacks

Most of you are aware of the limited number of snacks available to you while dieting. Here are a few suggestions for something a little different.

Marinated Vegetables: Cut carrots in quarters lengthwise. Take cauliflower and separate into flowerets. Take broccoli and separate into flowerets; cut the stems into 1-inch lengths. Cover cauliflower, broccoli, and carrots with boiling water for one minute. *Don't boil.* Just cover with boiling water, then drain. Put vegetables in a bowl and add diet Italian or French dressing. You can also add tomato wedges or some cherry tomatoes at this point. Marinate at least six hours. These make an excellent munch or can be used as a salad.

Baked Parsley: I've tried baked parsley for a snack. Don't laugh. It can be done. I got the idea from eating fried parsley, which I loved, but it has no place on a diet.

Wash and clean one bunch of parsley, pat dry, and separate. Spread in a lightly-oiled pan. Springle lightly with "crazy salt" or onion salt. Bake 15 to 20 minutes in a 350° oven until dry, but not brown, shaking occasionally. Cool. The taste will surprise you.

Gorp: Many teens are enthusiastic about a combination snack food called "gorp," which can be purchased in health food stores. They feel that this is so nutritious that they can eat unlimited amounts of it. After investigating the contents of gorp, I found it included dried fruit, coconut, nuts, and seeds. The average calorie count is about 400 to 500 per cup. Therefore, although gorp is nutritious, natural and healthy—it is not a good diet food.

There is a munch that is quite satisfying and has far less calories than gorp. A cup of this a day is about 100 calories (the same calories as an apple).

1 package straight pretzels (any size)
2 cups Shredded Wheat bits
2 cups Cheerios
2 cups plain popcorn
Onion salt
1 tbsp. imitation bacon-bits
1 tbsp. Worcestershire sause

Combine the onion salt and Worcestershire sauce and sprinkle over the mixture of popcorn, pretzels, and cereal. Heat in 250° oven for about one hour, stirring often. During the last half hour add one tablespoon of imitation bacon-bits.

Baked Potato Skins: When it comes to snacks, don't forget baked potato skins. Wash potatoes, peel them, and bake the skins in a lightly-oiled pan for 35 to 45 minutes at 350°. (Save the potatoes for the rest of the family.)

Soups

The first course of a meal can help fill you up and also add needed nutrients to your diet.

A cup of hot bouillon made from a cube can take the edge off your appetite. Even better is a can of tomato or vegetable juice, heated and served with some salted, unbuttered popcorn floating on the top.

A nice touch when you're serving a clear soup, and one which adds only a few calories to each portion, is making egg drop soup. Beat an egg with salt and pepper (and some chopped chives if you like), and stir it into 2 cans of boiling broth. Two cans and one egg will make enough soup for four persons, so you can treat your family to a surprise. You can also mix in a few fresh mushrooms, some chopped spinach, and even some chopped tomatoes. A teaspoon of soy sauce and you have something special

It's a good idea to cultivate new tastes on a diet. Many times you think that you can't possibly like something, but when you try it you think it's great. Something like that happened when I took my family to Spain several years ago. Certain things appeared on the menu constantly, and one of my sons, who was an extremely fussy eater, finally decided to try them because there wasn't anything else for him to eat. He ended up leaving Spain with a love for two or three dishes that he never would have tried in the United States.

One of these was a cold soup called Gazpacho. Gazpacho is a wonderful, low-calorie way to start a meal and can even serve as a whole meal. It is delicious and refreshing. The Spanish call it a "liquid salad."

Gazpacho (Salad Soup)

    1 cup finely-chopped, peeled tomato
    ½ cup finely-chopped green pepper, celery, and cucumber
    ¼ cup finely-chopped onion
    2 tsp. chopped parsley
    1 tsp. chopped chives
    1 small clove of garlic, minced
    2 to 3 tbsp. tarragon wine vinegar
    ½ tsp. salt
    ¼ tsp. black pepper
    1½ tsp. Worcestershire sauce
    2 cups tomato juice

Combine ingredients in a bowl, cover, and chill at least 4 hours. Serve in chilled cups with extra chopped vegetables and chopped hard-boiled egg. Serves 6.

For a little extra spark, instead of regular tomato juice use a spicy Bloody Mary mix and omit the pepper and Worcestershire sauce.

I was at a restaurant recently that served Gazpacho in green pepper cups. You didn't get much soup, but it really looked good.

Another soup that's fun to make comes from France. French cooking is not especially low-calorie, but I have tried to cut calories and still preserve the taste. You've probably seen this soup in restaurants, served in a crock and covered with bubbling cheese. Accompanied by a salad, it can serve as a whole meal.

French Onion Soup

4 large onions, sliced thin (1 onion for each serving)
1 tbsp. butter
2 cans condensed beef stock
1 can water
1 tsp. Worcestershire sauce
4 tbsp. grated Parmesan cheese
6 thin slices of small French bread (½" thick and toasted)
4 to 6 slices of Swiss cheese (¼" thick).

Cook onions in butter until tender and most of the water has been cooked out. (Be careful not to burn them, but be sure they are quite dry.) Add broth, water, Worcestershire sauce, and Parmesan cheese. Cover and simmer 20 minutes. Season with salt and pepper. Pour soup into ovenproof bowls until they are nearly full. Float 1 slice of toasted bread atop each. Cover each bowl with a thick slice of Swiss cheese. Place on foil and broil 4" from heat, until cheese starts to melt and turns golden. Serves 4.

Soup can be a great pick-me-up between meals and can often be used as a snack. Some of the instant soups that are no more than 80 calories (such as tomato or vegetable) are often useful on a cold day when you come home from school and are extremely hungry. In some of the diets, I've allowed you to take a cup of noncream soup instead of a fruit. One cup of shredded cabbage plus one can of stewed tomatoes adds a nice flavor to a plain vegetarian vegetable soup.

Sandwiches

Sandwiches are not necessarily a no-no in dieting. However, I prefer they be eaten for breakfast or lunch, and not for dinner. I also am always looking for different low-calorie ways to prepare them.

Sandwiches can be made in three ways. The first is open-faced. Use the thin-sliced or high-fiber bread, which saves you at least 20 to 30 calories a slice. Put the bread on the bottom and the filling on the top. This can be messy, but still tastes very good.

The second is a *reversewich*, in which you can use only solid fillings like cheese or cold meat. The cheese or meat is on the outside and one piece of bread is in the middle.

The third kind of sandwich uses interesting, low-calorie alternatives for bread. One is pita bread, a Syrian bread product that looks very much like a puffy flying saucer and is being touted for its low-calorie qualities. Actually, a very small pita is 80 calories, but it can be cut in half and both side filled with a variety of sandwich fillings—tuna fish, egg salad, and so on. The filling is limited because there is not much space in the pita bread. However, the bread is chewy and fun to eat.

Corn tacos, at 60 calories apiece, make a wonderful base for different kinds of sandwiches. Try one with chili, chopped tomato, lettuce, and cheese.

Half a bagel hollowed out (about 70 calories) can also be filled with tuna, crab meat salad, or any moist filling.

If you still insist on a real sandwich, the new thin-sliced breads or high-fiber breads at 45 calories a slice are certainly not going to damage anybody's diet.

The cleverest idea I've seen in a while is the "applewich." Core an apple and cut it crosswise into four layers. Fill it with cheese (at 100 calories an ounce), tuna, or one tablespoon of peanut butter (100 calories). Consider it an entire meal, easy to pack for lunch and quite different. This works with pears, also.

Cheese

Cheese makes a tasty appetizer. But my French cooking teacher always frowned on its use before a meal because, she said, it was too filling.

Cheese is a rich source of protein, although 73 percent of its calories are derived from fat. It is good as a primary food in dieting. But it is also excellent when used to enhance other foods. I like to grate it over meats, vegetables, or eggs. Cheese is so versatile it can be used in any number of ways.

1. *A Swiss cheese sandwich* on rye with hot mustard is a hearty, high-protein lunch.
2. *Cheese with fresh fruit* is a convenient way to carry one's lunch if no refrigeration is available. (Cheese should be eaten at room temperature anyway.)
3. *Fried cheese.* Heat a Teflon pan until it's quite hot, put in a slice of American cheese and just as it starts to melt and brown, flip it over and fry on the other side.
4. *Quiche.* Quiches are becoming very popular because they are easy to make, freeze, and reheat. Here is a simple version of a crustless quiche that I use when I want a quick meal.

Quiche à la Barbara _____

> 1 large onion,diced
> 1 tsp. salt
> 1 tbsp. butter
> 2 cups shredded Swiss cheese
> 2 cups nonfat milk
> 4 eggs
> ½ tsp. dry mustard
> 2 dashes Tabasco sauce

Sauté onion in butter until tender. Place on bottom of 8" square pan. Cover with shredded cheese. Combine eggs, milk, and other seasonings and pour over layer of onion and cheese. Bake in 350° oven for 35 minutes or until somewhat puffy. Cool for 10 minutes and slice into large squares.
Serves 6 to 8.

Eggs

Eggs are a marvelous diet food that are not fully appreciated by the dieter. They can be scrambled, poached, or soft-boiled. They can be made into omelets—plain or with bacon, cheese, ham, chives, and cream cheese. They become egg salad or deviled eggs quickly and easily.

When my kids were little I made them "gashouse eggs." Take the center out of a slice of bread, making a round hole in the middle. Drop the bread into a lightly greased pan and fry until it is slightly brown. Break the egg into the hole in the center of the bread and cook it until the white sets. Then you flip over both the egg and toast. It seems both the egg and the bread taste better this way.

Even eating plain hard-boiled eggs can be satisfying. Remember those colored Easter eggs? Hard-boiled eggs have the added advantage that they can be prepared ahead of time and eaten on the run.

One piece of advice: never eat an egg without pepper—it does unbelievable things to the flavor.

Deviled Eggs _____

> 2 eggs
> 1 tbsp. diet mayonnaise or diet dressing
> ¼ tsp. dry mustard
> 1 tsp. grated raw onion
> Salt
> Pepper
> Paprika (optional)

Hard-boil the eggs. (Always prick the middle of the bottom of the wide part with a needle before you put it into boiling water. This prevents the shell from cracking and centers the yolk of the egg. My favorite way of hard-boiling eggs is to plunge them into rapidly boiling water, let the water come back to a boil, turn off the heat, cover the pan, and let them sit for 20 minutes.) Shell the eggs, cut in half, and remove yolks. Mash the yolks with a fork and mix them with mayonnaise or dressing. Season with salt and pepper to taste, dry mustard, and onion. Fill the egg-white halves with the prepared yolks. Sprinkle with paprika and garnish as you wish with parsley, chives, or a slice of olive.

Other good seasonings for deviled eggs are Worcestershire sauce, Tabasco, chili sauce, and chopped bit of bacon.

Baked Eggs in Tomato Sauce

2 eggs
8 tbsp. tomato sauce
1 slice high-fiber bread (cut into small cubes)
2 tsp. grated Parmesan or Romano cheese
½ tsp. safflower oil
Salt
Pepper

Preheat oven to 350°. Use the oil to grease 2 ovenproof custard cups. Place 2 tablespoons tomato sauce on the bottom of each cup. Add half of the bread cubes, which have been toasted, to each cup. Break 1 raw egg over the bread cubes in each cup and cover the eggs with 2 more tablespoons of tomato sauce. Sprinkle 1 teaspoon of cheese on top of each cup and bake for 20 minutes.

Fish

According to that paragon of cooks, James Beard, fish should be broiled, baked, or poached 10 minutes per inch thickness. This formula works beautifully. In other words, if you want to broil a fish steak which is 1″ thick, preheat the broiler and put the fish on a pan covered with aluminum foil. Sprinkle the fish with lemon juice and a bit of oil or margarine and put it under the broiler for exactly 10 minutes. Serve the fish sprinkled with paprika and more lemon. Garnish with parsley.

To bake fish, preheat the oven to 425° to 450° before cooking your fish. Frozen fish must be cooked for twice as long as this formula suggests. Leftover cold fish is good the next day served in a salad with diet mayonnaise or salad dressing, chopped celery, onion, and pimentos.

I'm sure you've all heard fish is a brain food. Not so. The value of fish lies in the fact that it is high in protein, low in calories and usually low in fat.

Fish is not a naturally-popular food with most teen-agers. Tuna fish is an exception. Water-packed tuna (160 less calories than the oil-packed) is good plain or doused with wine vinegar, imitation bacon-bits, and a little hot pepper sauce. Even tuna salad made with 1 teaspoon of mayonnaise for each 3½ ounce can is acceptable. Person-ally, I like the idea of using plain water-packed tuna because it is dry and takes a lot of chewing and, therefore, seems more filling than tuna salad. You don't have to like many kinds of fish. You can have a very successful diet eating only tuna.

You might enjoy swordfish because the texture is much more like meat and it doesn't have a fish flavor.

Fish seasoned with margarine or lemon juice and baked in the oven for 7 to 10 minutes until it flakes easily makes a delicious low-calorie dish.

Always accompany fish with lemon. It sparks the flavor.

Fish dipped lightly in a seasoned flour and fried in a tablespoon of oil is not that fattening and might be a way you could learn to appreciate it.

I'd try not to eat a fish with bones because it always seems to traumatize people. My husband wouldn't eat fish for years because all he could remember was his mother serving him fish that was filled with sharp little bones that got stuck in his throat.

Maybe you would like this recipe:

Orange Fish

1 lb. filet, any white fish
2 tbsp. soy sauce
1 tbsp. ketchup
2 tbsp. frozen orange juice concentrate, thawed
1 clove garlic, finely chopped
1 tbsp. lemon juice

Combine all the ingredients in a baking dish. Dip any filet of white fish—sole, halibut—into the sauce. Cover completely and then, while lying in the sauce, bake at 350° for about 15 minutes until fish breaks easily with a fork. Serves 2 to 3.

No section on fish would be complete without mentioning seafood, which includes lobster, shrimp, crab meat, clams, scallops, and mussels.

A great many of these crustaceans, particularly lobster and shrimp, have become prohibitively expensive. However, for extravagant eating, one of the best low-calorie treats I can think of is this simple dish. Take medium- to large-sized shrimp, plunge them briefly into boiling water until they just turn pink (be careful not to overcook them), peel and serve with a spicy cocktail sauce made from Tabasco, ketchup, and horseradish. Delicious!

I don't like raw oysters or clams but their followers adore them. I think they improve incredibly with a small amount of cooking. Clams broiled briefly under a piece of bacon with a dusting of Parmesan cheese are delightful.

Beef

Beef has fallen into disfavor lately because of its high fat content and its high cost. However, even though red meat is being phased out of a lot of diets, I still find that most teen-agers enjoy it. Most beef is very easy to prepare. Steak is magnificent just broiled or charcoal-broiled, plain or brushed with marinade. If steak is too expensive, hamburgers are great, relatively inexpensive, and versatile. They can be eaten plain or topped with Swiss cheese, Cheddar cheese, bacon, chili, chopped onions, tomatoes, green peppers, and even a poached egg.

Chili is fun to eat, and it does not have to be fattening. It can be made without the beans. It's very high in protein and adds variety to a diet. Serve it by itself. There is no need to serve chili on rice or noodles.

Chili is simple to make and can be spicy or mild according to your taste buds.

Chili

1 pound lean ground meat
1 whole large onion, chopped
1 stalk celery, chopped
1 tbsp. corn oil
Salt
Pepper
Chili powder to taste (1 tbsp. to start)
1 small can red kidney beans (optional)
1 small can stewed tomatoes

Sauté and celery in oil until soft. Add ground beef and cook until red color has disappeared. Drain off fat. Add tomatoes, 1 tablespoon chili powder, ½ teaspoon salt, ¼ teaspoon pepper. Cook together over low heat for about 15 minutes or until mixture thickens. Pour into bowls and serve with tossed green salad. Makes between 3 and 4 servings, depending on your appetite.

Chili may also be used as a topping for hamburgers, hot dogs, or even string beans or zucchini squash.

Since ground meat will probably be one of the main ways you will be using beef, here are two other popular ways to prepare it.

Meatballs

Meatballs are very versatile. They go in different sauces—tomato, yogurt, mushroom, and others. They can be made small enough to be eaten as an appetizer or large enough to be a main course. They can be cooked ahead of time and reheated. Their flavor can be varied by the addition of different spices or different ingredients.

Basic Meat Balls

> 1 pound lean ground beef
> 2 tbsp. grated onion
> 1 tbsp. ketchup
> 1 tbsp. Parmesan cheese
> 1 egg
> 1 tbsp. chopped fresh parsley

Season the meat with salt and pepper, grated onion, ketchup, parsley, and Parmesan cheese. Add egg. If the mixture appears too loose, make crumbs from 1 slice of high-fiber bread and add until the mixture holds the shape of a ball. Shape into balls and bake in a 300° oven for 20 to 30 minutes (depending on size).
Serves 3 to 4 as main dish; 6 to 8 as appetizers.

The idea of baking meatballs instead of frying them saves calories. At this point, the cooked meatballs may be dropped into a spaghetti sauce (I'll give you a basic recipe for spaghetti sauce), chili sauce, canned cream soup (made with skim milk), or eaten plain.

You can change the taste of meatballs by adding different spices. If you want Italian meatballs, add ½ teaspoon of oregano per pound of beef. If you want a Mexican flavor, add 1 teaspoon to 1 tablespoon of chili powder per pound. If you want an Indian flavor, add 1 teaspoon curry powder and 1 tablespoon of yogurt to each pound of meat.

The same recipe for meatballs can be used for meat loaf. Just pack in a loaf pan and top it with ketchup. Bake 35 to 45 minutes in a 350° oven. Drain the fat from the pan as soon as you remove the meat loaf from the oven.

Another way to prepare ground beef is in stuffed green peppers.

Stuffed Green Peppers

4 large green peppers
½ cup cooked rice
1 pound ground beef
1 tbsp. minced onion
1 small can tomato sauce
2 tbsp. grated Cheddar cheese
Salt
Pepper

Core and seed peppers and drop them into a pot of boiling water to cook for about 10 minutes. Remove and drain. Mix ground beef, rice, onion, and ½ cup of tomato sauce. Season with salt and pepper and stuff the peppers with this mixture. Pour the balance of the tomato sauce into the bottom of the pan. Stand the filled peppers upright (you might have to cut the bottoms off to make them stand upright) and sprinkle with Cheddar cheese. Bake for about 30 minutes in a 350° oven until the beef is cooked.
Serves 4.

Tomato cases may be used in the same manner and may be made by cutting hollows in large unpeeled tomatoes, salting them, and inverting them to drain for 15 minutes. Tomatoes, however, tend to get soft during the cooking process and should be placed in greased custard cups to bake.

Flank Steak

This is a nice cut of beef because it has very little fat and is chewy, tasty, and filling. Spread it with 1 tablespoon of low-calorie Italian dressing, Worcestershire sauce, or barbecue sauce, and broil about 5 minutes on each side. Slice thinly on the diagonal (it makes it more tender). It makes a great meal and is delicious as a cold leftover, too. It also tastes good marinated with teriyaki or soy sauce and then charcoal-broiled on an outdoor grill.

Beef Kabobs

Kabobs refer to meat on a skewer—plain or alternated with vegetables or fruit (any kind), depending on your preference. Beef is usually used in kabobs, although lamb or chicken are delicious, also. One of the problems with kabobs is that when they are cooked on a skewer with vegetables, the vegetables cook at a different rate. When the meat is done, the vegetables may not be completely cooked. A cook named Bertha solved that problem for me. She skewered the meat and vegetables separately and allowed them to cook different lengths of time.

2 to 2½ pounds sirloin steak or good grade of round steak or tenderloin cut into 1½ inch cubes. Marinate in teriyaki sauce, soy sauce, diet French dressing, or barbecue sauce. Marinate small boiled onions, a large green pepper cut into chunks, fresh mushroom caps, and 1 box of cherry tomatoes. Drain marinade from vegetables and meat, and skewer separately. Broil the meat 3″ from the broiler, turning and brushing with marinade for about 12 to 14 minutes for rare beef. *Bake* the vegetables for 30 minutes at 350°. Time the baking of the vegetables with the broiling of the meat so they will be finished at the same time.

Chicken

My favorite diet food is chicken. It is low-calorie, readily available, economical, low in fat, and surprisingly versatile. Unfortunately, one of the easiest ways of cooking chicken is often neglected; that is, roasting it. Roasting is just another word for baking, and roasting a chicken imparts flavor and moistness that cannot be achieved by broiling. Ideally, a roaster should weigh between 3 and 4 pounds. The dieter dry-roasts poultry, using no additional butter or fat. There is a new gadget on the market—the chicken stands vertically to roast. It looks rather bizarre to open your oven and see a chicken standing on its end, but it keeps the bird from lying in fat and produces more even brownness.

Roasted Chicken ─────────────────────────────

> 1 whole chicken
> ½ lemon
> ½ medium onion
> 1 celery stalk
> 1 tsp. salt
> ½ tsp. pepper

Preheat oven to between 300° and 350°. Rinse the chicken under cool running water and dry thoroughly with paper towel. Rub inside and out with the side of a lemon. Season inside with salt and pepper and put onion and celery inside cavity to add flavor. Tie the legs together (any piece of white cord or thread will do), and close the neck with a toothpick. Place the chicken on a rack on a roasting pan, breast down, and bake in a 300° oven for 30 minutes per pound or a 350° oven for 20 minutes per pound. Turn breast up for last ½ hour of roasting. You can test for doneness by moving one of the legs up and down (if it moves easily, the chicken is done) or use a meat thermometer.

Poached Chicken Breasts

> 1 whole chicken breast, skinned, boned, and split
> 1 chicken bouillon cube
> 1 small piece of celery top
> ¼ onion
> ½ carrot
> 1½ cups water

Bring water to boil and drop in bouillon cube, celery, onion, and carrot. Simmer covered for about 10 minutes and then remove vegetables and insert chicken breast. Cover and keep water at a gentle simmer for about 20 minutes. Remove chicken and chill. Don't discard the bouillon used in cooking the chicken. It is a flavorful drink.
Serves 1 or 2.

In France these are known as "supreme de volailles," and they are indispensable for the dieter.

Following are just a few chicken recipes that will show you how different chicken can taste when prepared in different ways.

Apple-Glazed Chicken

> 2 chickens (3 pounds each), cut into pieces
> Salt
> Pepper
> 1 onion, finely minced
> 1 slice ginger root
> 1 cup apple juice
> 1 tbsp. lemon juice
> 1 tbsp. honey
> 1 small green apple, peeled and minced
> 2 to 3 red apples, cored and cut in eighths

Season chicken with salt and pepper. Lightly oil a 13″ × 9″ baking dish. Place chicken in pan, skin side up. Combine apple and lemon juices, minced onions, and ginger, and pour ¼ of it over chicken. Bake uncovered in 375° oven for 1 hour until golden (basting occasionally).

(One method of assessing how done a chicken breast is, is pricking it with a fork. If the juices run clear, then the chicken is done. If they run red, it is not.)

Add honey to the remaining juice, bring to a boil, and add minced apples. Dip the cored and peeled apples until they glaze, then take the chicken out of the pan, put the glazed apples around it, and spoon the rest of the juice over it. Do not take any sauce out of the saucepan, as a lot of fat from the chicken has collected there. Make sure the skin of the chicken is well-browned.
Serves 4 to 8.

Now for a little something with the Italian touch.

Chicken Cacciatore

2 whole chicken breasts, boned, split, and skinned
½ tsp. salt
⅛ tsp. pepper
1 tbsp. butter or margarine
1 small green pepper, cut into strips
½ cup chopped onion
½ diagonally sliced celery stalk
2 tomatoes, chopped
1 tbsp. fresh dill

Sprinkle chicken with salt and pepper. In medium skillet, melt butter and brown chicken on both sides. Remove from skillet. Add green pepper, onion, and celery. Cook vegetables until crisp and tender. Return chicken to skillet. Add tomatoes and dill. Cook over medium heat 30 minutes or until chicken is done.

Easy! Easy! Easy!
Serves 2 to 4.

Chicken Parmesan

4 chicken breasts with skin
Basic tomato sauce recipe (see Italian Food)
Grated Mozzarella cheese

Place chicken breasts, sprinkled with garlic salt, in 375° oven for 20 minutes until skin starts to brown. Then place 3 tablespoons basic tomato sauce over

each chicken breast and bake 10 minutes more. Sprinkle with Mozzarella cheese and cook until the cheese melts.
Serves 2 to 4.

The flavor of chicken can be changed remarkably with a marinade sauce, and one of the most popular of all marinade sauces is teriyaki, a mildly sweet form of soy sauce. Here is a recipe for Polynesian Teriyaki.

Polynesian Teriyaki

> ½ cup soy sauce
> 1 tbsp. salad oil
> 1 tbsp. molasses
> 1 tsp. ginger root, minced
> 2 tsp. dry mustard
> 4 cloves garlic, minced
> 2 pounds chicken parts (breasts, thighs, or drumsticks)

Combine the first 6 ingredients. Add chicken to marinade, stirring to coat. Let stand at least 2 hours at room temperature. Broil 4″ from heat for about 5 to 7 minutes on each side if it is a breast, and about 10 to 12 minutes on each side if it is a thigh or leg. Brush frequently with marinade. Test for doneness by piercing with a fork to see if the juice runs clear.
Serves 6 to 8.

Feeling French? Try . . .

Cordon Bleu Chicken

> 3 chicken breasts, split (about 12 ounces each)
> 6 thin slices lean cooked ham
> 6 thin slices Swiss cheese
> Fresh minced parsley
> Instant garlic powder
> 1 tsp. salt
> ¼ tsp. pepper
> ⅓ cup fine, dry, bread crumbs
> 2 tsp. vegetable oil

Skin and bone the chicken breasts. Flatten slightly with a wooden mallet or the edge of a plate. Place a ham and a cheese slice on each chicken piece; sprinkle with the minced parsley, garlic powder, salt, and pepper. Roll up chicken to enclose ham and cheese; secure with wooden picks. Blend bread crumbs with oil and place in a flat plate. Press each chicken roll into the mixture to coat

lightly. Place on a *nonstick* baking sheet. Bake in moderate 350° oven for 35 minutes or until chicken is tender.
Serves 6.

And now a great salad using chicken:

Cobb Salad

> ½ large head lettuce, shredded
> 2 chicken breasts, cooked, chilled, and diced
> 2 medium tomatoes, diced
> 3 hard-boiled eggs, chopped
> 8 slices cooked bacon, crisp and crumbled
> ¾ cup crumbled blue cheese
> 1 medium avocado, halved, peeled, and cut in wedges
> 1 small stalk French endive
> 1 tbsp. snipped chives
> ½ cup diet French dressing

Place shredded lettuce in large salad bowl. Over lettuce, arrange a row each of chicken, tomato, egg, bacon, and cheese. Tuck in avocado wedges and endive leaves to garnish. Sprinkle with chives. Toss with French dressing.
Serves 2 to 4.

Foods of the World

One way to vary menus is to copy from the different countries of the world. Some of the most familiar and best loved foods come from Italy, France, China, and Mexico. The dieter should get ideas from all these countries.

Italian Food

It is a popular assumption that Italian food is very fattening, so many dieters avoid it. Actually, I've had some of my best diet meals in an Italian restaurant, but you must know how to order. I order half a broiled chicken with plain spaghetti *sauce* on the side, a large green salad with oil and vinegar on the side, and perhaps a vegetable sautéed with garlic and oil. I'll feel like I've had a real Italian meal, and if you notice, it includes no spaghetti or bread.

Sometimes I start my Italian meal with an antipasto. Antipasto means *before* the spaghetti, but since you won't be eating the spaghetti, your antipasto could be a whole meal. It usually consists of cold, lean meats, marinated vegetables (such as mushrooms, artichokes, and eggplant), hard-boiled eggs, cheese, and perhaps some roasted Italian-style peppers.

If you want to make an antipasto yourself, it's easy. Be sure you drain the oil off any prepared marinated vegetables, or if you marinate them yourself, make the marinade (which is a sauce that flavors the vegetables) with ½ cup oil and ½ cup vinegar. Serve an antipasto on a full dinner-size plate so it becomes the whole meal. You need only your imagination to make a good one, and here is a sample one you might like to try.

First, you line the bottom of a plate with leafy green lettuce. Do *not* use iceberg lettuce. Marinate raw mushrooms (in diet dressing or your own marinade) in the refrigerator overnight, and place a few on the plate. Buy some very thinly-sliced Italian ham or use regular baked ham. Roll it up like a cigarette and add wedges of salami, pepperoni, or Italian sausage to the plate. Garnish with cherry tomatoes and peppers, hard-boiled eggs, and celery stuffed with lowfat cottage cheese that has been flavored with garlic salt. Get some provolone cheese (it comes in a round shape), and cut half moons to put around the outside of the plate. You can even serve the antipasto with bread sticks and still have a diet meal.

Two things that Americans find very characteristic about Italian foods are the tomato sauce and garlic. In order to know what goes into the tomato sauce, you should make it yourself. Otherwise, you could be the victim of sugar, preservatives, and more fat than you need. I have a recipe given to my by my aunt for a super tomato sauce. It can be stored in the refrigerator for several weeks or it can be frozen in little containers and used as needed.

Basic Tomato Sauce _____

    1 large can stewed tomatoes
    2 large cans tomato sauce
    1 small can tomato paste
    1 large can Italian-style stewed tomatoes
    1 bay leaf
    ½ tsp. oregano
    1 tsp. basil
    2 cloves garlic

3 tbsp. Parmesan cheese
1 slice green pepper
½ carrot
Salt
Pepper

Cook all the ingredients together for one hour. Remove the carrot and the green pepper and bay leaf. Season to taste with salt and pepper. (I'll bet you're wondering why there's a carrot in the tomato sauce; tomato sauce can have a very sharp flavor, and the carrot is a natural sweetener.)

Where are you going to use your tomato sauce? Over the meatballs and vegetables; or try this recipe for lasagna without the noodles.

Noodleless Lasagna

3 cups lowfat cottage cheese (drained well), beaten with 4 eggs
4 heaping tbsp. Parmesan cheese
1 pound lean ground beef
1 or 2 cloves garlic, minced
Salt
Pepper
2 cups shredded Mozzarella cheese
2 cups basic tomato sauce

Brown beef with garlic in a Teflon pan and drain well. Season with salt and pepper. Take an 8″ × 8″ square baking dish, and layer browned meat, Mozzarella cheese, basic tomato sauce, and cottage cheese mixture in the dish. Repeat layers. Top with thin slices of Mozzarella cheese and bake 45 minutes at 350° until set. Allow to stand 15 minutes before serving.
Serves 6 to 8.

Love the taste of pizza? Then it must have been upsetting to have seen all the calories in one piece. There are ways to get the pizza *taste* without all the calories.

One way is to take eggplant, slice it crosswise, and broil it until it's slightly soft. Top it with one tablespoon of basic tomato sauce, shredded Mozzarella cheese, a pinch of oregano, and bake until cheese melts. This could be a low-calorie pizza or, in layers, eggplant Parmesan.

You may also use frozen tortillas (60 calories each) as a pizza crust. Separate them, put them on a greased pan, and bake them for about 10 minutes at 350° until crisp and firm. Top with one tablespoon of basic tomato sauce, Mozzarella cheese, and oregano, and heat until the cheese melts. If you want something fancier, you may add mushrooms, onions, or green pepper.

One-half of an English muffin, although not as low in calories, can also be used as a pizza crust. Or try this . . .

Tomato Slice Pizza

> 2 large, firm tomatoes
> ½ small can sliced mushrooms, drained
> 2 slices Mozzarella cheese
> 1 tsp. oregano
> Salt
> Garlic

Preheat oven to 350°. Cut 4 thick slices from the tomatoes, place slices on a cookie sheet that has been greased with oil. Divide the mushrooms among the tomatoes, and place half of the Mozzarella on top of each. Sprinkle with oregano and bake for 3 minutes until cheese is melted. Turn on broiler and let cheese brown lightly. Season with salt and garlic.
Serves 2.

You really should save spaghetti for when you're maintaining your weight, although ½ cup is allowed on the Carefree Diet. On most weight-loss diets, though, it's okay to put spaghetti sauce on other foods such as French-style string beans, zucchini, squash, shredded lettuce, baked meatballs, and chicken.

Mexican Food

Mexican food can add variety to your diet without adding a lot of calories. The flat corn tortilla, covered with a mixture of meat, shredded lettuce, chopped tomatoes, shredded Monterey Jack cheese, chopped onions, and perhaps some chopped green chilies, is a dieter's dream.

Filling for Tacos

> 1 pound ground beef
> 2 cloves of garlic
> 2 tbsp. basic tomato sauce
> 1 tbsp. chili powder or taco seasoning
> Salt
> Pepper

Sauté ground beef with garlic in a Teflon pan and drain off all oil. Add the basic tomato sauce and chili powder or taco seasoning mix. Salt and pepper to taste. Cook about 10 to 15 minutes, mashing down with a fork to try and make the mixture as fine as possible. Take 2 tablespoons of mixture and put it on a corn tortilla. Sprinkle with the toppings you want.
Serves 4 to 6.

Enchiladas make a relatively low-calorie and dramatic main course. In the enchilada, the frozen (not the crisp) tortilla is used so it can be thawed and rolled around the filling.

Enchiladas _____

Sauce
3 medium onions
1 tsp. olive oil
2 one-pound cans crushed tomatoes
2 cups tomato sauce
2 tbsp. finely-chopped, canned, green chilies
1 packet artificial sweetener
1 tsp. salt

Filling
¾ pound ground beef, lean
2 small cloves garlic, minced
1 tsp. olive oil
½ cup sliced green onion
3 tbsp. chopped ripe olives
2 tsp. chili powder
Flat tortillas

Sauce. Cook chopped onions in olive oil until tender. Add next 5 ingredients. Simmer uncovered for 45 minutes.

Filling. Cook beef and garlic in 1 teaspoon of olive oil. Add the next 3 ingredients. Simmer 10 minutes. Thaw tortillas. Fill with 2 tablespoons of meat mixture. Roll up. Arrange enchiladas in a heat-proof platter. Cover with sauce and cheese. Bake at 350° for about 25 minutes.
Serves 6.

Chinese Food

I will devote more space to Chinese cooking because it is delicious, healthy, and very much in vogue at the present time. If you keep away from the deep frying and go easy on the rice and noodles, you may adapt any Chinese recipe to your diet and perhaps you will evolve into a skilled Chinese cook, complete with wok, cleaver, and chopsticks.

Chinese food, as I was introduced to it as a child, was a thick, gooey, overcooked mess called chow mein, which was spooned over rice and under fried noodles. How glad I am that it bears little or no resemblance to Chinese food as it really is.

Some of the things that make Chinese cooking great for diets is that the meat quantities are kept to a minimum, which is economical and lower in saturated fat, and the vegetables are crisp and filling. One can use any combination of meat, fish, and vegetables, and the basic formula is the same. The meat is usually sliced thin and marinated in a combination soy sauce and corn starch. This marinade not only flavors the meat or the seafood, but also tenderizes it. Then you cut the desired vegetables into small uniform pieces (Chinese like symmetry). The meat and vegetables are cooked separately and briefly in a small amount of oil in a process called stir-frying. The meat is cooked until it just loses its redness (except for pork), and the vegetables are cooked until they are just crisp and tender. The two are combined at the last minute.

Texture, color, and shape are very important in Chinese cooking. Texture refers to the feel of the food as you chew it. Textures can be rubbery, soft, silky, crisp, and stringy.

Remember, in Chinese cooking you must *not* overcook the vegetables. They should be crunchy. That is one reason why Chinese cooking has to be done at the last minute. Foods can be sliced or chopped ahead of time, but the actual cooking should be done immediately before you eat.

The most important cooking tool needed to prepare food in the Chinese style is the *wok*. A wok is a cooking pan shaped like an upside-down coolie hat and is extremely useful in recipes for both deep-oil frying and stir-frying. The electric woks are Teflon-coated, temperature-controlled, and allow you to use less oil than you would ordinarily need. They are also attractive enough to use as a serving dish at the table.

A sharp knife is invaluable for all the slicing, chopping, and mincing you must do. Even if you are lucky enough to have a food processer that cuts, shreds, and chops, a sharp knife is still quite important.

Chinese vegetables are delightful, and you should acquaint yourself with them. They add much color and crunch to the food.

Bamboo shoots are available in cans. They come in chunks or sliced thinly. Remove the bamboo shoots from the can and rinse them in cold water. If you don't use a whole can, store the rest in a small plastic bag and freeze them. They have a mild flavor and a granular consistency rather like a pear.

Fresh *bean sprouts* should be used whenever available, as they are far superior to the canned ones. Three cups of fresh, uncooked bean sprouts equal ½ pound; 1½ cups of cooked bean sprouts equal 1 pound. Clean fresh sprouts by putting them in a bowl of cold water, then drain them. They should be cooked very briefly to preserve their crispness. Canned bean sprouts, on the other hand, have no crispness at all and taste slightly medicinal. To improve them, rinse them several times with cold water and briefly immerse them in chicken stock.

Water chestnuts are found whole, in cans, and you slice them the way you want them. They have no flavor, but they're interesting because of their crunchy texture.

The Chinese used *dried mushrooms,* which have an excellent flavor, but you must get used to them. When I first tasted Chinese mushrooms, I found them overpowering. Now I enjoy their unusual flavor and chewy texture, even in American dishes. They come dried in cellophane packages. To prepare them, soak them in hot water for 20 minutes. Squeeze the water out of them, and then they are ready for chopping and slicing.

Other Chinese vegetables include *bok choy* (Chinese cabbage), *pea pods, bean curd* (from soy beans), and the gummy *black fungus.*

The Chinese have many different flavorings for their food. In this country we are familiar with *soy sauce,* but equally important are *hoisin sauce, plum sauce, oyster sauce,* and *ginger root.* Fresh ginger root is now available in many stores. It looks just like a root. It is peeled and sliced thin or chopped and added to recipes. It has a much more subtle taste than the dried and powdered ginger that we are used to.

There were many recipes I could have included in this section, but I have included the most simple and most familiar. Once your taste buds have been stimulated, you might want to go on to more exotic dishes.

Chow Mein

    1 pound pork, beef, shrimp, or chicken, cut into thin strips
    2 cups onions, sliced
    1 cup bamboo shoots, drained
    2 tsp. oil
    3 dried mushrooms, soaked in hot water and chopped
    3 cups fresh bean sprouts
    1 tsp. fresh ginger root, chopped
    1 tsp. sugar
    1 tbsp. corn starch
    2 tbsp. soy sauce
    ½ cup soup stock

Fry the meat in 1 teaspoon of peanut oil until it loses its red color. Remove the meat from the pan. In the same pan, sauté mushrooms, bamboo shoots, and onions in 1 teaspoon of oil for 1 or 2 minutes and add to the meat. Then, without using any more oil, sauté the bean sprouts and the chopped ginger root. Return meat and vegetables to pan. Add a mixture of sugar, corn starch, soy sauce, and chicken stock. Stir until thickened. This should take about 2 or 3 minutes.
Serves 4 to 6.

The basic Chinese stir-fried dish can be varied with many vegetables. One pound of meat is marinated with 1 tablespoon of corn starch and 1 tablespoon of soy sauce. This is allowed to stand for 15 to 20 minutes. Then using a maximum of 1 tablespoon of oil, stir-fry the meat with any vegetable you desire.

Beef and Onions

    1 pound beef, sliced thin
    2 tbsp. soy sauce
    1 tbsp. corn starch
    1 tbsp. oil
    3 cups thin-sliced onions
    1 tsp. sugar

Marinate beef in soy sauce and corn starch. Heat oil in wok. Fry beef until it loses its red color. Remove beef from wok and add the thinly-sliced onions. Stir-fry for about 2 to 3 minutes. Return beef to wok with remainder of soy sauce marinade and sugar, and allow to simmer for 2 minutes.
Serves 4 to 6.

You may use this basic formula with snow peas, cauliflower, green peppers, broccoli, or asparagus, or change beef to chicken or seafood.

When you get to the point in your diet where rice is allowed, Chinese fried rice happens to make an excellent main course and is quite filling. It requires no accompaniment other than a cup of tea and a fresh fruit for dessert.

Fried Rice

    1 tbsp. peanut oil
    2 cups onions
    1 can or 3 cups fresh bean sprouts
    2 cups cold, cooked rice
    2 eggs
    1 tsp. *thick* soy sauce
    ½ tsp. salt
    2 cups chopped cooked meat or seafood

Heat oil in pan and fry the onions and bean sprouts until slightly limp. Add 2 cups of cold, cooked rice. Stir-fry. Add to the mixture 2 eggs that have been mixed with thick soy sauce and salt. Sauté until the eggs are set, and then you may add any leftover meat or fish.
Serves 4.

Vegetables can all taste better—both American and Chinese types—cooked in a Chinese fashion.

Chinese Zucchini

    2 tbsp. oil
    4 cups zucchini, cut into julienne strips
    1 large onion, chopped
    Salt
    Pepper
    1 tbsp. soy sauce
    2 cups fresh, sliced mushrooms
    ½ cup fresh bean sprouts
    Sesame seeds (optional)
    Bamboo shoots

Heat oil in wok. Add zucchini and onions and fry for 2 minutes. Remove from wok and add bamboo shoots and bean sprouts. Stir-fry for 2 more minutes.

Add soy sauce. Remove from heat. Combine zucchini with other vegetables. Sprinkle with 1 teaspoon of sesame seeds, if desired.
Serves 4 to 6.

This can be done with broccoli, asparagus, cauliflower, green pepper, and eggplant. The firmer vegetables, like broccoli and asparagus, should be covered with boiling water for 1 minute and drained before stir-frying.

Here's a Chinese dish that incorporates a variety of vegetables:

Chow-Vegetables

> 1 head bok choy (Chinese cabbage), sliced in 1″ pieces
> ½ cup carrots, sliced thin
> 2 cups fresh Chinese pea pods, blanched for 2 minutes in boiling water
> 1 tbsp. peanut oil
> 1 cup sliced mushrooms
> 3 cups fresh bean sprouts
> 1 basket of cherry tomatoes
> ½ cup oyster sauce
> 2 packets artificial sweetener
> ½ cup soy sauce
> Salt and pepper

Sauté cabbage, carrots, and pea pods until just slightly cooked in the oil. Add mushrooms, bean sprouts, tomatoes. Simmer 1 or 2 minutes, taking care the vegetables do not overcook and remain crisp and crunchy. Make a sauce of ½ cup oyster sauce, 2 packets artificial sweetener, ½ cup soy sauce, salt and pepper. Blend all ingredients thoroughly and flavor the mixed vegetables with this sauce.
Serves 6 to 8.

Want a Chinese dish that won't kill your calories for the day? Try egg foo yung.

Egg Foo Yung

> 1 cup bean sprouts, fresh if possible (or ½ can)
> 1 tbsp. each of green onion, chopped bamboo shoots, finely-chopped water chestnuts
> 3 mushrooms, chopped (optional)
> Salt
> 4 eggs

Combine all ingredients and mix well. Heat 1 teaspoon of salad oil in a Teflon skillet and spoon in ⅓ cup of egg mixture to form each cake. Fry over high heat until puffed and delicately browned, turning once. Stack several cakes for each serving. Makes 6 cakes.

Salads

Salads are not just lettuce and tomatoes. They can be exciting adventures. Instead of putting them in a bowl and mixing them, sometimes it's nice to get a round platter, cover it with shredded lettuce, and see what raw vegetables you can add. You can make a ring of cucumbers, cherry tomatoes, green peppers, and sprinkle some thinly cut onion over all.

If you want to make a Greek salad, add feta cheese (a mild, pleasant soft cheese), black olives, and dress with one tablespoon of olive oil and lemon juice.

If you want to make the same basic salad into an Italian one, sprinkle with chopped anchovies, cut scallions, ½ teaspoon of oregano, and dress with wine or garlic vinegar and one tablespoon of olive oil.

For a Chinese touch, add bean sprouts, chopped water chestnuts or sesame seeds, and dress with one tablespoon of peanut oil and rice vinegar.

Go Mexican by adding chopped green chilies and shredded Monterey Jack cheese.

For just a plain American salad, use as is, but add hard-boiled egg wedges, celery, carrots, and low-calorie dressing.

Some salad ideas are:

1. Sliced tomatoes, cucumbers, and onions with scallions and diet dressing sprinkled over all.
2. Thinly sliced cucumbers combined with sliced onions and a dressing made with 1 cup vinegar, ½ cup of water, and a packet of sugar substitute. Allow it to marinate for 3 to 4 hours.
3. If you like yogurt, try thinly sliced cucumber and onions and fresh dill added to ½ pint of plain yogurt.
4. There was a salad that I ate in a little restaurant in Pennsylvania that I particularly liked. It was simple but interesting. Fill a bowl with shredded lettuce. Then grate separately 2 ounces Cheddar cheese, 2 ounces baked ham, 2 ounces white meat chicken, and 2 carrots. Layer each ingredient over the lettuce and serve with low-calorie Italian dressing. Because the meats and vegetable are grated, their flavors mix beautifully with the lettuce. Great!

If you have a salad without lettuce, it's good to store it in the refrigerator to allow the flavors to mingle with each other and the dressing. If you have lettuce in a salad, however, or any other kind of leafy green, allowing it to stand *after* you have poured dressing on it will only make it wilt. You should toss salads with lettuce immediately before you are going to eat them.

Don't forget the fruit salad. A fruit salad can be used as a meal and is often a good dieting alternative for meat. Try to use only fresh fruits in season. Don't worry if they are high or low in calories, and don't peel apples or pears. Cut into good size chunks; it gives a salad more eye appeal. Add bananas or strawberries to a fruit salad if you expect to eat it that day. Be sure to add a squirt of lemon juice to keep the fruits from discoloring and ¼ cup of orange juice for moistening. Serve, as is, with absolutely no dressing. A good fruit salad is not to be disguised.

Cantaloupe Salad

    1 ripe cantaloupe
    1½ cups lowfat cottage cheese
    1 small can pineapple wedges in own juice, drained

Chill cantaloupe and slice into 3 even sections removing seeds. Remove rind. Mix cottage cheese and pineapple bits. Place melon slice on a lettuce leaf on individual plates, and fill center with ⅓ of the cottage cheese mixture.

Pineapple Boats

    1 ripe pineapple
    Apples
    Pears
    Tangerines
    Mandarin oranges

Choose a ripe pineapple (it'll have a delightful odor), and cut off top and bottom with a sharp knife. Stand the pineapple on its end and cut lengthwise into 4 pieces. Cut down and remove the core from each piece with a grapefruit knife. With the grapefruit knife, scoop under the meat, separating from the skin, but not removing it. Then cut the meat into 1″ sections. Remove every other piece (put these aside to eat at some other time), and replace with wedges of apples or pears, skin side up, or tangerine or mandarin orange sections. Place on a lettuce leaf.

Melon Bowl

> 1 small ripe watermelon
> 1 ripe cantaloupe, peeled, seeded, and cut into wedges
> 3 peaches, pitted, skinned, and sliced
> 1 pineapple, rind removed, cored, and cut into wedges
> Small bunch green grapes, stemmed
> ½ pound red cherries, pitted and halved
> 1 small bottle diet lemon-lime drink
> Lemon juice

Lay the watermelon on its side and slice off top third. Scoop pulp out of melon and remove as many pits as you can while cutting into chunks. Mix in large bowl with balance of fruit, a squirt of lemon juice, and the lemon-lime drink. Put fruit back into bottom part of melon and decorate with mint leaves or parsley.
Serves 12 to 14.

There is a salad that my grandmother used to serve all the time when I was growing up. I thought it was the most delicious thing imaginable, and I never was a cottage cheese fan.

Russian Salad

> 1 pint lowfat cottage cheese
> 1 tomato, chopped
> 6 radishes, sliced across the grain
> ½ green pepper, cubed
> 1 stalk of celery, sliced
> ½ cucumber, sliced thinly
> ¼ cup chopped onion

Mix all ingredients together and season with salt and pepper. If you prefer a more creamy consistency, add a tablespoon of yogurt or mix in a tablespoon of lowfat sour cream. You can omit any vegetables you don't like, or add any vegetables that you do like. Serve on a lettuce leaf.
Serves 2.

Asparagus Salad

> Canned or fresh asparagus
> Pimento
> Red or green pepper
> Hard-boiled egg
> 1 tsp. mustard

This can double as a salad or a vegetable. For each person, place 3 or 4 spears of chilled and cooked, fresh or canned asparagus on a lettuce leaf, crossing them with a slice of pimento or green or red pepper. Sprinkle with half a chopped hard-boiled egg. Serve this with diet Italian dressing that has been mixed with garlic, artificial sweetener, and a teaspoon of mustard.

I enjoy meat in a salad. Most people know the traditional Chef's Salad, in which salad greens are topped with a combination of ham, tongue, salami, roast beef, and cheese. But here is a different salad that uses chicken.

Mesa Salad

> 1 bed of fresh pale green Bibb lettuce (Bibb lettuce is that soft, tender lettuce, as opposed to the crisp iceberg lettuce)
> Chicken breast
> Chinese pea pods
> Sliced water chestnuts
> Chilled bean sprouts
> Tomato wedges
> Mandarin oranges

Place slivers of chilled, poached chicken breast next to whole Chinese pea pods, sliced water chestnuts, and chilled bean sprouts. Garnish with 2 or 3 tomato wedges, and center with a small amount of mandarin oranges. Serve with a spicy diet French dressing. This is a single serving.

In California, salad is often served as a first course before the main dish and is a filling and important part of the meal. Always remember that a good part of a salad's special appeal depends upon fresh, colorful, chilled ingredients and crunchy, crisp textures.

Fun-City Salad

> Lettuce
> Green pepper
> Tomatoes
> Red onions
> Carrots, grated
> Apple with skin, chopped
> Celery, chopped
> Cucumber sticks
> Sliced radishes
> Green vegetable

For each person place a few flat lettuce leaves on a chilled salad plate. Quarter the plate with green pepper strips and in one section place thinly sliced or chopped tomato and red onion; place grated carrots in the second section; chopped apple and celery in the third; and the fourth might have cucumber sticks, some sliced radishes, or a chilled green vegetable. Serve bowls of diet and regular dressings separately.

Everyone's favorite!

Spinach Salad

1 cellophane package fresh spinach or 1 pound loose
4 scallions using part of the green stem
1 hard-boiled egg, yolk and white, chopped
2 slices bacon, crisply fried, drained, and crumbled
1 can artichokes, drained (optional)
6 fresh mushrooms, sliced thinly (optional)

Dressing: ⅓ cup wine vinegar
⅓ cup vegetable oil
½ tsp. dry mustard
⅓ cup water
Salt
Pepper

Carefully wash and remove stems from spinach. Dry leaves thoroughly and place in salad bowl. Sprinkle with scallions, chopped egg, bacon, artichokes, and mushrooms. Mix the ingredients for the dressing, pour into the salad bowl, and toss until leaves are fairly coated. This salad may be served with 1 can of drained mandarin orange slices and 1 tablespoon of sliced almonds instead of egg, bacon, and mushrooms.
Serves 3 to 4.

There are just too many delicious salads in this world to begin to list them here. Just keep some of these combinations in mind:

1. The washed leaves of a bunch of watercress, combined with a bunch of radishes, sliced and chilled.
2. Lettuce, sliced cucumbers, shredded green pepper, diced celery, sliced green onions, and sliced tomatoes with a little garlic added.
3. Tomato stuffed with tuna, egg, or crab-meat salad or cottage cheese.
4. Lettuce, hard-boiled eggs, drained tuna, cold sliced green beans, and cold sliced boiled potatoes with 1 or 2 black olives for garnish make a Salad Nicoise. This is usually served as a main luncheon dish, is

always garnished with red onion slices, and has an oil and vinegar dressing.

5. Sliced or slivered boiled ham, Swiss cheese, roast beef, turkey, salami, and a garnish of a slice or two of hard-boiled egg on a bed of lettuce is the ever popular Chef's Salad.

6. Cabbage, onion, carrot, green pepper, all grated and flavored with tomato slices and celery seed, dressed lightly with oil and vinegar, and seasoned with salt and pepper makes a wonderful slaw. You may also add dill or caraway seeds.

7. Two or three varieties of lettuce (iceberg, romaine, Bibb, escarole leaf, curly red) with fresh sliced tomatoes and a pinch of basil.

8. Romaine lettuce, anchovies, croutons, Parmesan cheese, and Caesar dressing make a wonderful Caesar Salad.

9. Chilled or sliced raw mushrooms, boiled and sliced frozen artichoke hearts, sliced water chestnuts, chilled bean sprouts, and bamboo shoots may all be added to any salad.

10. Artificial bacon-bits or real crisp bacon crumbled, grated Parmesan or Romano cheese, or shredded Cheddar cheese all enhance the flavor of a salad.

11. And, finally, remember that any of the familiar cooked vegetables you are used to eating hot may be chilled and added to a salad. These include: whole green and Italian beans, beets, pea pods, zucchini, brussels sprouts, and broccoli.

Vegetables

Most teen-agers don't seem to like cooked vegetables, except for corn and peas. This is a shame, because in cooked vegetables you can get a variety of food tastes and a lot of bulk for a small number of calories.

How can cooked vegetables be made more appealing to you? Buy the fresh vegetables. Cut them in different ways. You'll be surprised how the shape alters the texture and the flavor. Take the carrot, for instance. Cut it in sticks. Cut it on the cross-grain. Shred it. Now cook it. Cook it crisp and tender (Chinese style) and add salt and pepper. Cook it soft and add butter, salt, and pepper. Add some lemon and artificial sugar for a sweet and sour taste.

Most vegetables improve enormously by being steamed rather than boiled. Try out lots of herbs and seasonings, and see what appeals to you. Also, don't forget that a squeeze of lemon will make any vegetable taste better. If you love butter, but hate vegetables, by all means start out by putting butter on your vegetables, and then gradually use less as you learn to appreciate the taste of the vegetables alone.

Stir-frying makes vegetables more appealing.

Another interesting way to prepare vegetables is in combination. Anyone who has eaten in a school cafeteria knows about succotash, which is lima beans and corn. Well, it tastes better when thin sticks of carrots and celery are steamed together with green and wax beans, zucchini, or yellow squash (don't peel the squash, just rub it well). You'll be surprised at how these colors and tastes complement one another. Don't forget to use fresh ground pepper on them.

Make plain steamed carrots appealing by dropping them, once they are cooked, into orange juice to which a teaspoon of brown sugar has been added. Heat the ingredients together.

I'm going to make an example of two unpopular vegetables—the *most* unpopular vegetables—and ask you to try and see if you can develop a taste for them because they are both so low in calories.

The first one is mushrooms. Mushrooms can grow all year round in almost any site, so there is a constant crop flow, and *yet* the supply *cannot* keep up with the demand. If you aren't eating mushrooms, you are missing a great low-calorie food (20 calories a cup). In order to get used to them, try the canned variety first. Drain them, and mix with another vegetable you like. There is a steak house in our city that started serving a combination of onions and mushrooms. Mushroom popularity zoomed. After you have combined them with something you like, taste them straight. Next time you are *hungry,* open a small can and enjoy. Now you are ready for the real thing—fresh mushrooms. Mushrooms are to be wiped or lightly washed and the ends of the stems trimmed off. Melt a teaspoon of butter, slice the mushrooms, and sauté them until they are soft. Put on top of a steak or hamburger or combine with onions so you don't get overwhelmed by the taste. Or you can try them in an omelet or in your basic spaghetti sauce. Sauté (fry in a small amount of butter) one cup of mushrooms, add one cup basic spaghetti sauce, and serve over hamburger, string beans, or spaghetti squash.

Now try baking them. Put mushrooms into a greased pan. Sprinkle them with onion or garlic salt and bake for about 20 minutes. Chewy!

If you are lucky enough to have some large mushrooms, detach the stems from the caps, chop the stems up, and sauté them in butter with some chopped celery. Mix with crabmeat or ground hamburger and crumbs made from one slice of high-fiber bread. Stuff the caps with this mixture, sprinkle with Parmesan cheese, and bake for 25 minutes.

Finally, you are ready for raw mushrooms. *Raw* mushrooms fill you up better because they contain such a large percentage of water, which is lost when you cook them. First slice them, then add to your favorite salad. The vinegar in the salad dressing actually cooks the mushrooms because they are so delicate.

Now you're ready for the real mushroom test. Wash, dry, and trim firm mushrooms. Sprinkle with crazy salt, diet salad dressing, imitation bacon bits, or eat straight. When you can do this, you have become a real mushroom fan.

Stuffed Mushrooms

    12 large mushrooms
    1 small celery stalk, chopped
    1 small can water-packed tuna (3½ oz.) drained
    3 tbsp. grated Parmesan cheese
    ½ lemon, squeezed
    1 tsp. vegetable oil
    Salt
    Pepper
    ¼ tsp. garlic powder

Wash the mushrooms and dry thoroughly. Separate caps from stems. Place the caps hollow side up in a greased baking dish and sprinkle with lemon juice. Chop the stems and sauté them with onion and celery in your nonstick skillet, using just a bit of oil. Mix in the drained tuna, salt, pepper, garlic powder, and squeeze of lemon. Fill the mushroom caps with the cooked mixture. Sprinkle with cheese and bake for about 15 minutes at 350°.
Serves 3.

In any of my travels, the most hated food that I have come across is spinach. While it doesn't build muscle, it is a marvelous source of vitamin A and potassium and has only 42 calories per cup cooked.

The way to start appreciating spinach is to start eating it *raw* and *fresh,* unlike mushrooms, and progress to the cooked stage. Initially, fresh spinach has a gritty taste, so be sure you wash it well. Place a few chopped spinach leaves in a regular salad. It's a pretty contrast to the light green of iceberg lettuce. Then try a spinach salad on its own, with bacon, chopped hard-boiled eggs, scallions, and Italian dressing or mandarin oranges and slivered almonds with a sweet, low-calorie Russian dressing. This is a start, and as soon as you get more daring try heating spinach briefly in clear chicken soup to wilt it, and serve Chinese style with some scallions on the top.

Now you are ready for cooked spinach. Cook a bunch of spinach, drain it, mix with 2 eggs, 1 minced onion, salt and pepper, ¼ cup of skim milk. Pour into greased custard cups and bake for 30 minutes at 350°. Once you've grown accustomed to the taste, you can switch from fresh to frozen spinach, which is quite good. If you really want to enjoy spinach, *don't* try the canned variety.

Another way to make vegetables taste better is to make a soufflé, which is a very fluffy mixture made with eggs. This dish uses either spinach or broccoli and is also a good main dish for the vegetarian.

Spinach Soufflé

1 package frozen chopped broccoli or 1 package frozen chopped spinach
2 eggs, slightly beaten
1 tbsp. all-purpose flour
1 cup shredded cheese (any type you like)
1 cup lowfat cottage cheese
½ tsp. salt
½ tsp. pepper

Cook the frozen vegetables according to package instructions. Drain well, combine with eggs and flour, and mix until smooth. Stir in remaining ingredients. Pour into glass casserole and bake for 25 to 30 minutes at 350°. Serves 4 to 6.

Here's a good recipe for broiled tomatoes, used especially when tomatoes are plentiful.

Broiled Tomatoes

2 large tomatoes, cut in slices crosswise, ½" thick
2 tbsp. diet mayonnaise
4 tbsp. grated Parmesan cheese
4 tbsp. green onion, minced and sautéed
2 tbsp. parsley.

Combine diet mayonnaise, cheese, green onion, and parsley. Spread on tomatoes. Place into preheated broiler for 2 to 3 minutes until lightly browned. Serves 4 to 6.

There are two foods all dieters should investigate. One is tofu, a soybean protein (or bean curd), which is relatively low in fat. If you've ever had hot and sour soup in Chinese restaurants, those creamy strips floating around in it are tofu. It comes in fresh squares stored in plastic containers or preserved in cans. Some of my patients slice it, broil it, and eat it plain. It doesn't really have that much flavor, but it will take on the flavor of anything that it's cooked with.

The other interesting food is spaghetti squash. It looks like a yellow football and comes in various sizes. If you're lucky enough to have a microwave oven, puncture some holes in the squash with a fork, and bake it on high for 10 to 15 minutes. If you use a regular oven, spaghetti squash requires about 45 minutes cooking time. You bake it in its skin, slice it open, clean out the seeds, and you find a delicate yellow squash that separates into strands that look like spaghetti. I eat it with Parmesan cheese, salt, and pepper. After eating half a spaghetti squash, which is about 50 calories, I am quite full. A whole spaghetti squash almost does me in. It can be used as a basis for spaghetti sauce, or it can be served with just butter or margarine, salt, and pepper. It also adapts to almost any topping you want to put on it.

Eggplant is another good vegetable to learn to eat. It also combines well with so many things—tomato sauce, cheese, onions, for examples.

Eggplant Deluxe

1 medium size eggplant, cut in half
1 No. 2 can tomatoes, drained and mashed
2 strips of bacon
1 small can mushrooms, sliced and drained
1 small onion, minced
1 slice high-fiber bread, crumbled
¼ green pepper, minced
1 slice Mozzarella or Cheddar cheese, grated
1 tsp. oil
Lemon juice
Salt
Pepper
Garlic powder

Sauté bacon slices until crisp. Discard bacon grease and drain bacon on paper toweling. Break into pieces and set aside. Scoop out pulp of the eggplant and chop, leaving shells about ¼″ thick. Squeeze lemon over the shells so they won't discolor. Sauté pulp, onion, peppers, and celery in nonstick skillet in which oil

has been heated for about 1 minute. Cover pan and simmer for another 7 minutes. Mix with onion, canned tomatoes, mushrooms, and bacon. Season with salt and pepper and fill eggplant shells with this mixture. Sprinkle tops with crumbs and cheese and place in pan with 1 or 2 tablespoons of water. Bake about 20 minutes at 350°
Serves 4.

One of my favorite foods is sauerkraut, and I wish you'd taste it, hot or cold. It has few calories, is good to munch anytime, and seems to satisfy a craving for something substantial when you're on a diet. Here is how I prepare it for a hot dish.

Sauerkraut _____

> 1 No. 2 can sauerkraut
> 1 can beef bouillon
> ½ onion, grated
> 1 tbsp. caraway seeds

Drain sauerkraut and place in a pan with bouillon and onion. Heat together to boiling, lower heat, and simmer, covered, for 20 minutes. Before serving, sprinkle with caraway seeds.

If you really don't think you can tolerate sauerkraut, try it piled on a foot-long hot dog with mustard and onion, and you *will* become a fan.

Desserts

I don't care what anyone says; desserts simply don't go well when dieting. I think all the time and effort one puts into a fancy, low-calorie dessert is wasted. The best diet desserts are fresh fruits in season: watermelon, strawberries, blueberries, peaches, pears, cherries in the spring and summer; oranges and grapefruit in the winter; apples in the fall. All can be eaten by the dieter and enjoyed.

I have often used blueberries and strawberries to make low-calorie sauces. I take a pint of blueberries, heat them briefly until they release their juices, add a tablespoon of Wondra flour and a tablespoon of lemon juice, and 3 packets of low-calorie sweetener. This makes a slightly thick sauce you can use over a lemon sherbet. It also goes well with cantaloupe.

The only other desserts dieters should be concerned with are sherbet, ice milk, angel food cake, pound cake, gelatin dessert, frozen custard, low-calorie custards, and yogurts and puddings made with skim milk. Commercial pound-cake slices are only 100 calories. You can have a low-calorie strawberry shortcake. Ice milk, ranging anywhere from 110 to 140 calories a scoop, is also a good occasional dessert, as is frozen yogurt and frozen custard. Vanilla wafers, between 20 and 30 calories a wafer, are a possibility if you can stop at one, two, or three wafers and not eat the whole box.

Another sweet you might want to try is angel food cake, which has comparatively few calories and can be purchased ready-made in the supermarket.

Once you get used to the idea that dessert does not necessarily have to be sweet, try munching on a sliver of cheese with a piece of fruit. That is how Europeans end their meals, and it is a most satisfactory way to do it. You will notice trays with a broad selection of natural, unprocessed cheeses in fine restaurants. Well, it would be wasteful and expensive to have six or seven cheeses on hand in your refrigerator, but you can afford one or two. Start with some of the more common cheeses like Cheddar and Swiss, then go on to Edam, Gouda, Havarti, Muenster, Port Salud, and the like. Try a small amount of each, one at a time. Experiment. From these you can branch out to others. Try the imports and stay with hard cheese rather than the soft, runny type, which is usually made with lots of cream. Always remember that cheese should be served at room temperature and tasted and savored rather than gulped. Just a sliver or two combined with a nice tart apple or a juicy pear make a great dessert.

As for your guests, you might try orange ambrosia. In your prettiest glass bowl, layer thin slices of naval oranges with shredded coconut. Sprinkle with a small amount of powdered sugar and refrigerate for a few hours. Or try:

Pears or Peaches With Fruit Purée

Peel, halve, and poach ripe pears or peaches in boiling water which has been flavored with lemon juice, 3 packets sugar substitute, and ½ teaspoon vanilla. Simmer until fruit is tender. Drain and chill. Defrost one package of frozen strawberries or raspberries and purée in a blender or mash through a sieve. Spoon over pears or peaches and serve sprinkled with a few chopped almonds.

Frozen Peaches

At the height of the peach season next summer, buy several pounds of this delicious fruit. Rinse and peel. This is easily done by spearing each peach on a fork and holding it in boiling water for 10 seconds. The skin can be slipped off as though by magic. (You can try this with tomatoes, too.) Halve and pit the fruit. Pack it into freezer boxes. Pour diluted frozen orange juice over fruit to within ½″ of the top. Cover and freeze. (These are absolutely delicious defrosted for dessert or used in a salad especially when fresh peaches are out of season.)

By the way, here are a few recipes for dishes included in the vegetarian diet section (Chapter 13).

Total Rice

Mix together in a 2-quart casserole 3 cups of cooked rice, ¼ cup chopped parsley, 1 cup grated Cheddar cheese, 1 cup chopped onions, 4 tablespoons chopped green pepper, 1 minced clove garlic. Blend and mix into rice 1 can (14½ ounces) of evaporated skim milk, 2 eggs, beaten, 1 to 2 tablespoons vegetable oil, ½ teaspoon salt, ½ teaspoon pepper, and 2 tablespoons lemon juice. Sprinkle with parsley and bake at 350° for 45 minutes until set.
Serves 4 to 6.

Carrot Casserole

Cook 12 sliced carrots until crisp tender. Make a sauce of 1 large chopped onion sautéed in 1 tablespoon margarine and 2 tablespoons flour, 2 cups skim milk, ½ teaspoon salt, ¼ teaspoon pepper, 2 teaspoons dry mustard. Measure and put aside 1½ cups buttered bread crumbs, ½ pound grated Cheddar cheese. Arrange layers of carrots, cheese, and crumbs. Pour sauce over and bake at 350° for 45 minutes.
Serves 4 to 6.

Bean Soup

Brown 1 chopped onion in 1 tablespoon butter, add 2 quarts of cold water and 2 cups lentils or other dry beans. Bring to boil, cover, and simmer for about 2½ hours. Add 3 sliced carrots, 3 chopped celery stalks with leaves, 1 teaspoon basil, 1 cup tomatoes, salt and pepper to taste. Continue simmering, covered, until vegetables are tender. Serve with grated cheese on top.
Serves 8.

21

Some Things You Want to Know

In my travels, I've collected hundreds of questions from teen-age girls. I tried to pick the most common. If I missed yours, drop me a line.

Will Dieting Make My Skin Better?
This is a controversial area, but the consensus of opinion seems to be *no.* Skin tone and color are as much a part of heredity as a glowing smile, pink cheeks, and sparkling eyes.

While it is true that a poor diet can cause pale skin (from anemia), dull eyes (from vitamin deficiency), and a dull smile (from general neglect), you would have to be quite malnourished to show these signs. Some very healthy girls are pale and sallow and need blush for that pink-cheeked look.

Pimples have nothing to do with diet. When your hormones begin to work at the start of adolescence, several glands begin to secrete oil. If they secrete too much oil too fast, your pores become plugged up, and the result is pimples. You can scrub the excess oil out of pores, but the real trouble is from *within;* it's not related to chocolate, nuts, eggs, or fat.

Rashes are another matter. Pimple-like skin rashes can be the result of certain kinds of food sensitivity. Chocolate and citrus fruits are the biggest offenders.

Incidentally, you cannot tell anything about people's sex lives or habits of masturbation by the number of pimples they have on their faces.

Will Dieting Make My Teeth Better?

I have a son who stopped drinking milk at the age of two, never ate cheese, and doesn't have a cavity in his mouth. He has naturally good teeth.

I lived on milk until I was six, loved dairy products, and don't have a tooth in my mouth without a filling. Again, short of absolute malnutrition, the quality of the enamel on your teeth is often something you are born with. Neglect can make the best enamel wear down, but the neglect has to be substantial.

The sparkling smiles you see in commercials are due to natural tooth color or caps (yes, models do get their teeth capped). Not all people have white teeth. You can brush twenty times a day, but teeth come in shades of white, yellow, and gray (and all combinations thereof). Don't despair. Dentists can now paint your enamel to make it look whiter.

Dieting can indirectly help your teeth if it causes you to decrease the amount of sugar you consume. When the enamel on a tooth isn't sturdy, nothing promotes tooth decay like a high-sugar diet. The biggest culprits are candy and cake, which get lodged next to the base of the tooth. There, fermentation initiates the breakdown of enamel, which makes the tooth more liable to decay.

Gums are now receiving a lot of attention. People used to think they had no function other than picture frames for teeth. Now dentists have discovered that healthy gums help retain natural teeth longer. Gums do respond to stimulation, good nutrition, and massage.

Flossing has become a national pastime and, if you have to put something in your mouth, it's a great alternative to eating. Flossing is moving a waxed thread in and out between your teeth to stimulate your gums. You can floss 3 to 4 minutes daily. Spread it into four one-minute sessions if you are doing it in place of eating.

Do They Have a Pill to Melt Fat?

Don't I wish! No, the only pills to help dieters are appetite depressants, which are of limited usefulness.

The most exciting thing I have heard about lately isn't a pill, but a cooking oil that tastes good, can be used in salads and for frying, and doesn't get absorbed, so you get zero calories.

Will Being Overweight Affect My Health?

Interestingly, most girls can handle 20 to 30 pounds of excess weight without it affecting their health. This is because women are designed to carry extra weight when they're pregnant. However, as childbearing years come to a close, excess weight begins to affect the physical well-being of females much more dramatically.

When you are younger, excess weight can create problems like rashes between your legs and under your breasts—annoying, but not dangerous. Also, you are more prone to get small skin infections in the folds of the groin or under your arms.

Actually, in females, obesity is more of a life-*spoiling* disease than a life-*threatening* disease, but it can make it *easier* for you to develop or make it more difficult to control these dangerous conditions.

1. *High blood pressure,* which can lead to a stroke or heart attack.
2. *Diabetes,* which is a gradual exhaustion of your insulin supply, the result of pushing your insulin to the limits.
3. *Arthritis,* which can be aggravated by stress on the back and knees.

Scientists have now suggested that obesity increases your chances of getting certain types of estrogen-related cancer. This is because fat has a role in the conversion of pre-estrogen into estrogen. Therefore, if a cancer is dependent on estrogen—as are breast, uterine, and ovarian cancer—then fat could play a role in stimulating it.

In addition to these life-threatening problems, being heavy at your young age slows you down and can rob you of a lot of enjoyment in everyday activities. Your expected life span is 77 years—your body has a long way to go. Fat wears you out before your time.

If I Eat Only Healthy Food, Will I Lose Weight?

I think it's good to eat healthy food. Raisins, nuts, seeds, dried fruits, and legumes are terrific—they are loaded with vitamins and good taste. But they are also loaded with calories. Fresh vegetables, fresh fruit, eggs, cheese, and meat are also healthy foods, but they don't have as many calories.

There is a difference between healthy food and dietary food. A weight-loss diet should be healthy, but not all healthy diets produce weight loss. There are some females who are on a very healthy diet and don't lose one ounce, gaining weight just as if they were eating junk.

Does My Body Know When I Need Certain Foods?

The body has no natural intelligence about anything except fluids: if your water intake is decreased, your body will tell your brain that it needs a drink. Natural intelligence stops there.

If you feel tired and think you need sugar, it's not your body talking, but your mind. You learned early in life that sugar is a fast source of energy. Some people crave oranges and say it's because they need vitamin C. Why doesn't the body direct you to eat other vitamin-C-rich foods, such as tomatoes, yellow squash, or papayas? It is because you have learned that orange juice has lots of vitamin C, and you *like the taste*. Even those cravings for *chocolate* before your period are usually just general carbohydrate cravings, caused by changes in fluid balance. People choose chocolate specifically because they love chocolate.

Will Vitamins Make Me Hungry?
No. That is an old wives' tale. Vitamins sometimes make you feel better, and when people who have been sick start feeling better, they regain their appetites. In healthy people there is no reason to think that vitamins increase appetite.

There are no vitamins that *decrease* appetite either, except in toxic doses. Some initial findings suggest that reducing the levels of certain minerals in the body, expecially zinc, can curb appetite. But this research is in the experimental stage and has little application for teen-agers.

Can I Take Too Many Vitamins?
Yes. If you noticed in our vitamin section, the fat-soluble vitamins—A, D, E, and K—have dangerous and toxic side effects, so they should only be taken in prescribed doses. I also have patients that eat too many carrots, and they actually develop yellow palms. This is more alarming than it is serious. If you stop the carrots, the color will disappear.

Will Exercise Make Me Hungry?
No. As I said in the exercise chapter—and I'll say it again because it's important—exercise is great with dieting because it *decreases* your appetite, keeps you busy and away from food, and makes you look thinner, even if the scale does not show a weight loss. In fact, if you get uncontrollable hunger urges, I recommend that you run up and down the stairs five to ten times. (But don't tell your parents to do the same—they may get heart attacks.)

While I'm on the subject of exercise, what about the exercise fitness centers that are cropping up all over the country? Sign nothing unless you read the fine print. Sign nothing unless you are prepared to pay a healthy chunk of money. Your parents can't get you out of these kinds of contracts, so if you can't pay, they will have to. If you understand the financial and time commitments of these centers, and you feel that it is the only way you can exercise, by all means join. As you know, I prefer the aerobic exercises to calisthenics, but both have their place in a weight-loss program. Most of the centers also offer diet programs.

Passive massage machines are worthless anyway. From the old "relaxicizers" that used to shock your muscles into moving, to the present massage machines that pound you black and blue, they really don't help you lose weight.

What Determines the Size of My Breasts?

Heredity determines breast size. Breast size is not determined by how much food you eat, unless it is so little or so much that starvation or enormous obesity result. In cases of starvation, as in anorexia nervosa, the breasts often don't develop. This is due to the resulting slowdown of all hormonal functions, including estrogen production.

There are many thin teen-agers who wear a size C cup; on the other hand, there are obese girls who wear a size A.

It's difficult to predict the final size of one's breasts in the early teens. Normal breast development in girls goes through five stages, taking anywhere from one-and-a-half to eight years. By the time most girls have had their first period, they still have not completed the process. As a matter of fact, your periods may start at the age of 12, and your breasts may not be completely developed until you are 18 or 20. On the other hand, don't be alarmed that you are going to be enormous if you are well-developed by age 13—you might have already completed your growth.

Exercise does *not* influence the size of breasts, nor does it help sagging. Breasts are just skin, fat, connective tissue, and glands. There is no muscle there. If you sag, your skin is not sufficient to hold you up.

However, exercise *can* affect your posture, which has a lot to do with how your breasts stand out. Exercise can also affect the proportions of the rest of your body; if you reduce the size of your hips and waist, your breasts will look bigger by comparison.

Breasts will respond to hormonal stimulation. Since birth control pills are a form of hormonal stimulation, girls who take them might notice a small increase in their breast size. Pregnancy also causes breast enlargement. Part of this is caused by growth of the milk glands, and the other part is hormonally-distributed fat. Many young women talk about how flat-chested they were until they got pregnant and finally developed a bosom.

You are going to be teased about your breasts whether they are large or small. Sometimes boys accidentally or purposely bump into them. Pay no attention. No matter how you feel about them now, they make your clothes look better and your body anatomically interesting, and they will prove very useful to you if you decide to have children.

Can I Selectively Lose Weight in Certain Parts of My Body?

You tend to lose weight evenly all over, not from the place where you need to lose it. That's why your face may look drawn, even in the middle of a nutritious, well-balanced, weight-loss diet. You have less fat in your face, so when you lose a few layers, it really shows.

The last places on your body to lose are the ones with the most fat. Most females have a pear-shaped build—heavier on the bottom. A few are ice cream cones—top-heavy. However, most figure problems in girls are with legs, hips, and rear. Exercise alone will not take care of these because if there is an adequate amount of fat everywhere else, where is the fat going to go?

However, with specific hip exercises—leg rolls and side leg lifts—there is a slight possibility that with increased movement of those muscles, more blood is circulated to that area. Some people maintain that fat in those areas is preferentially carried away.

Of all exercise, jogging does the best job, since most of the motion occurs from the waist down. However, spot exercises won't hurt, and they make you feel like you are doing something.

How Come My Dress Is Getting Loose and I'm Not Losing Any Weight?

Fat is constantly being shifted around. If, you lose ten pounds in two weeks and then hold for the next six weeks, your figure will keep changing. Your hips, legs, and stomach will keep getting smaller; so much so that the clothes that fit you after the first two weeks of the diet are now baggy, but you haven't lost one extra pound. You are *redistributing*.

Remember, females have a layer of subcutaneous (under the skin) fat. This layer is constantly being reduced by dieting. The upper part of your body becomes more depleted than the lower part, because there is usually less fat above the waist. So in order to even out this layer, fat migrates from areas where there is too much to areas where there is less. In other words, after weight loss, the body attempts to normalize itself.

The migration of fat is a slow, slow process that doesn't happen when you are in the midst of a weight-reduction diet. After the diet, the fat has a chance to move around. I always say you lose from the head down and redistribute from the knees up.

Should I Take Up Smoking to Lose Weight?

No! No! No! Do you know what happens when eaters take up smoking? They eat *and* smoke. Then they have *double* trouble. Cigarettes, unless they are candy-coated, will never replace food in the lives of people who like to eat, any more than chewing gum will replace food. How many of you chew gum and still eat?

Many people are afraid to give up smoking because they might *gain* weight, and often they do put on a few pounds. This is because nicotine acts as a very mild appetite depressant, and, depending on the number of packs smoked, probably does increase one's basal metabolic rate (bodily consumption of oxygen) slightly. However, after a person has "dried out" for a few weeks, these physiological side effects disappear.

Some people also feel the emotional need to put something in their mouths. This can be satisfied by carrot and celery sticks cut into cigarette-size pieces. Unlike the overweight, the smoker does not need to put carbohydrates into her mouth.

If you are worried about gaining weight, attempt to diet at the same time you are quitting cigarettes. If you can maintain your weight, it will be a victory. If you do gain, you should still be happy about quitting smoking.

Is Alcohol Fattening?

Alcohol is a totally different kind of nutrient. It isn't a protein, carbohydrate, or a fat. It is called ethanol. It contains 7 calories per gram and burns quite rapidly. Because it is in the bloodstream within a few minutes after it is ingested, it is a rapid source of energy.

Alcohol supplies easy calories so that stored fat is not needed. Therefore, it slows down weight loss. There is nothing sadder than an overweight who likes to drink. That is the worst of both worlds.

Most overeaters enjoy good taste, so if they drink, they usually have banana daquiris, apricot sours, or sombreros—alcoholic drinks that are so heavy on sugar, fruit, and cream that the alcohol is a minor ingredient. These drinks are murder for your weight, containing more than 300 calories each. Other drinks are high, too: an average cocktail is 150 calories, beer 150 calories, and dry wine 100 calories for a 3½ ounce glass.

Drinking does something else besides add extra calories; it clouds good judgment and makes you more relaxed about what you are doing. You develop an "I don't give a damn, why not take a taste?" attitude that is quite dangerous to your diet.

You must decide either to eat your calories *or* drink them. Liquid or solids, they are still calories! Alcohol is nothing but empty calories, so if you choose to drink, you are depriving your body of essential nutrients.

I would like to add a word about drinking as a social obligation. I have adult patients who feel pressured to drink booze when they go out for a business lunch. That is as absurd as being pressured to eat. You don't have to drink to make anybody feel good. If you don't want to and if you don't like the taste, don't!

If some of your friends take you to a beer and pizza place, just order a tall glass of water or a plain soda with ice, and nurse it all night. Beer drinking will add nothing to the evening except calories. The exception to this is a lite beer that has less calories than even a soda—so have one glass, if you feel you must. Also, if you know you are going out that night, and will be drinking, skip dessert.

Will Pot-Smoking Hurt My Weight?

Pot or marijuana smoking is a fact of life, legal or illegal. I am not taking any moral or political position on it except to recognize that its use in our high schools and colleges is *not* uncommon.

My concern is its relation to weight gain. Like all smoking, it has no calories in itself, but it does interesting things to the smoker's appetite. As the height of the effects of the drug start to wear off, kids get overcome with what is popularly known as the "munchies," an intense craving for food. The "munchies" can only be satisfied with carbohydrates like candy, crackers, or popcorn. It even hits kids who do not usually get turned on to sweets. Like alcohol, it clouds your judgment and makes it easier to give in to certain impulses—like eating. In the course of a weight-loss diet, it can be devastating.

Most of my teen-ager patients do not smoke marijuana. There are certain aspects of the overweight personality that do not enjoy the marijuana experience. They are often a little more conservative than girls of normal weight and are simply afraid to try it. And besides ... they get their highs from food.

If you do have a weight problem and you also smoke pot, you are asking for trouble. But you can take the following precautions. Have plain, unbuttered popcorn with salt available. Even if you stuff down two or three cups, you can't do much harm.

Or tell yourself before you smoke that when you get the "munchies," you will eat only raw vegetables, dill pickles, or, at worst, little pretzel sticks. If you firmly imprint this message in your pre-conscious, it is usually possible for you to direct your food urges even under the influence of the drug.

Can Dieting Affect My Period?
Yes. No. Sometimes. Funny answer? Funny subject. I know girls who weigh 250 pounds and have their periods regularly every 28 days. I also know girls who become 10 pounds overweight and start skipping periods.

Periods respond to diet, stress, depression, and change of environment (going away to college is a good way to make periods irregular). Anorexics stop having periods because their fat gets below a critical level.

During the initial phase of your periods—the first two or three years—they are often irregular anyway. Losing weight can make them farther apart or closer together. If your periods are *too* far apart, you may have another problem.

Toni was a charming teen-ager who loved to eat, and her weight regularly shot up and down. She could lose or gain 50 pounds in a summer. She left my office in June after losing 50 pounds and returned in September with 60 pounds back. She weighed 210 pounds. She also stated that her periods were irregular, which they had been before she lost weight. She came to my office several times, couldn't get her act together, and lost no weight.

A few days after Toni's last visit, I received a phone call from the hospital emergency room. "Your patient, Toni P., came into the emergency room at 7:00 P. M. and immediately delivered a 7-pound baby boy," I was told. "Her mother fainted on the spot!"

After that experience, I take very careful menstrual histories whether the girls are 12 or 20. If they are old enough to get periods, then they are old enough to get pregnant, and this must always be considered when evaluating the cause of a missed period.

If periods are coming too frequently (every two to three weeks), this should be investigated also. The main problem here is too much blood loss, which could result in anemia. It is often due to a mild hormonal imbalance created by dieting. This is usually not serious.

Many girls complain to me that losing weight makes menstrual cramps more severe. This is because when you are fat you often do not ovulate. Ovulation occurs when an egg comes from the ovary to be fertilized. When it is not fertilized, you have your menstrual period. That is called an *ovulatory cycle*.

Sometimes when girls gain weight, their hormone balance is off and no egg comes from the ovary. That is called an *anovulatory cycle*. Losing weight can cause you to ovulate more regularly and simply, and ovulatory cycles give you more cramps.

Dieting can definitely help what we call "premenstrual tension," the "blues and blahs" of the last days before your period. This tension is due to fluid retention, which can actually alter your mood. When you are on a diet, you reduce your carbohydrate intake and retain less fluid, so miserable "menstrual moods" are not as severe.

Will Birth Control Pills Make Me Gain Weight?
If you have a tendency to be heavy, they certainly will! If you are thin, you might put on a few pounds of water weight, which you can take care of by decreasing your salt or carbohydrate intake for a few days.

If you have a weight problem, birth control pills can make it 10 percent easier for you to convert food into fat, which means you could gain weight. That means that if you have been maintaining your weight on 2,000 calories per day and you start taking the birth control pill, you will have to cut your calories by 10 percent—or 200 calories—to 1,800 calories, just to maintain the same weight.

If you wish to diet while on the pill, subtract 400 calories from your *new* maintenance level in order to lose one pound per week.

Even though it makes weight loss more difficult, taking birth control pills is better than taking a chance on getting pregnant. At least dieting offers no moral, religious, or economic hassles. So if you plan to have regular or semiregular intercourse, take the pill and cut back to the appropriate caloric level, or else expend more calories in exercise.

How Did I Get Stretch Marks and How Do I Get Rid of Them?

Stretch marks, or *stria,* are those funny purple wiggly lines you see on your breasts, hips, abdomen, and tops of the legs. They are the result of your body growing faster than your skin. They develop during periods of high hormonal stimulation like adolescence or pregnancy. Stretch marks represent the rupture of the elastic fibers in the skin, much like a rubber band that has been pulled too tightly and is no longer elastic.

These do not go away. Don't waste your money on fancy oils or creams. The purple color will fade eventually, and they will become light silver. Then you won't notice them as much.

How can you prevent them? Prevent large weight gains at times of high hormonal stimulation, like the one you are going through now.

However, sometimes you don't have to gain large amounts. of weight—your breasts and hips can suddenly round out, leaving marks. I have seen many thin girls who developed stretch marks in this way.

Some people take small amounts of zinc (10 milligrams per day) to increase skin elasticity, but I'm not sure it helps, and it might increase your appetite.

What Is Cellulite?

A few years ago a popular exercise book was published about the ugly "puckering" on the tops of women's thighs, which the authors named "cellulite." Although it is most common in older women, cellulite can also be seen in some overweight teen-agers. It was supposed to be an inflammation of fat, which required specific diets and exercises to cure.

Cellulite aroused so much interest that two teams of scientists set out to determine exactly what it was. What they found out was extremely interesting.

Cellulite is not an abnormal disease state, but a hormonal type of fat deposition on female thighs. Fat on the top of female legs is distributed in little pouches. When you get an excess amount, it pops out of the top like too much popcorn in a brown paper bag. If your skin is not tight, due to aging or poor quality, those fat bumps or the dimples between them become prominent.

The cures include diet to lose the fat and exercise to firm the thigh muscles. Enough exercise can flatten the fat between muscle and skin. Firm massage, along with weight loss, can help reduce the little pockets sooner because it gets rid of water that is trapped in the spaces between the fat.

Hand massage is fine—you don't have to be wrapped in any plastic or pounded on by any machine. Just put the palms of your hands flat against the sides of your thigh above the knees. Firmly press while sliding your hands up toward the top of the thigh. Repeat this about 10 times on each leg.

Cellulite probably isn't a problem to you, even if you are overweight, because you have firm skin; but if it is, dieting, exercise, and massage should make it disappear. If you absolutely hate the way it looks while you are reducing, wear stockings with shorts or tennis dresses (sheer heel and toe, please). Many people do that. Then, even if your thighs and legs are heavy, they aren't bumpy.

How Should I Dress While I Am Dieting?

It's a lot easier to be chubby now because designers of junior dresses cut them somewhat fuller below the waist.

When you are on a diet, *buy as few clothes as possible*. Make sure that what you buy will *look as nice as possible* for *as long as possible*.

First, analyze your body. Are your arms huge? Then wear long sleeves or no sleeves. There is nothing more unflattering then short sleeves on fat arms.

Is your neck fat? Don't wear high, round collars. V-necks or low ovals make your neck look longer.

Are your breasts huge? Then avoid clinging T-shirt materials that outline them.

You have no waistline? Don't wear a two-piece dress with a tight waistband. Wear a two-piece dress that has a long overblouse; it will give you an elongated look.

Huge hips? Avoid gathered skirts.

Fat tops of legs? No tight skirts.

Thick ankles? No ballet slippers or thin little heels. Wear platforms with as much heel as your mother will allow. Chunky heels make ankles look thinner.

Pants look terrible on most heavy girls, catching them at the worst part of their anatomy—the tops of their legs, their hips, and their rear ends. But the most important thing is that pants are *totally impractical when you* are losing weight. They look baggy even when you lose small amounts of weight. Forget about them while you are on a diet.

You will get the most service out of several jumpers with blouses and shirts. They can either be tent type A-lines, which flair out at the bottom without a belt, or full dresses where the belt is optional (as you develop a waistline, you can start belting them).

The smock style, which is gathered over the bosom and falls straight, is a great look for the overweight girl, provided your bust isn't too big. The wraparound skirt looks good, also.

All these styles will last through *20 to 30 pounds* and just look better as you get thinner. When you purchase dresses, T-shirts, or blouses, buy one that *just* fits, not one that fits comfortably. Elasticized waistbands are marvelous for the overweight. The only problem is that as much as they stretch on the way down, they also stretch on the way up.

Also, pay attention to your hair style. Remember, a full face should have a somewhat simple but *full* hairdo. Don't have your hair cropped short when you are at your heaviest. Use your hair to soften your face, but don't be too fussy or cutesy either. I have a 250-pound patient who has the new curly look, and she looks like a fat little Orphan Annie doll.

Can I Get Too Thin?

The Duchess of Windsor was credited as saying, "A woman can't be too rich or too thin." If you are healthy and eating well-balanced meals, it is difficult to get too thin. If you are starving yourself for the sake of beauty (and *you* say it's beauty) to the point where you have no energy and no appetite, then you are too thin.

I used to think that patients who complained about getting colds and other illnesses while they were dieting were looking for an excuse to stop the diet. Now, I believe there is a definite connection between immunity to disease and nutrition. If you are shortchanging your nutrition, there is no question that you can get too thin.

Is Overweight Always Unpopular With Boys?

Unless overweight girls are socially withdrawn, most of them have boyfriends who don't mind that they have a weight problem. The overweight girls who don't have boyfriends are putting out nonverbal messages that say, "I'm really inferior because I'm overweight."

The girls who exude confidence even though they might be heavy, especially 20 to 30 pounds overweight, don't seem to have any social problems at the high school level. Girls who are 40 or more pounds overweight have many more social problems.

What Is the Yo-Yo Syndrome?

The Yo-Yo Syndrome consists of a formal weight loss followed by a rapid weight gain. It happens like this: after several months, a girl finishes a successful diet. A month later, she has regained all her weight. Obviously, after she ended her diet, she returned to the same eating patterns that made her fat in the first place.

Is it bad for you to yo-yo? Yes! It is harder to lose weight after you've repeated this pattern a number of times. It seems that the fat cells become more resistant to being broken down the more times they are expanded. Also, there is a theory that more fat is deposited on the inside of the arteries when you lose and gain weight constantly.

It takes longer for the body to start losing the second time around, and even longer the third and fourth. Remember your first successful diet and how amazing the weight loss was? Then you regained weight and tried to go on the same diet again, but the weight loss was much slower.

Constant yo-yoing also causes you to develop a psychological defeat pattern. Many girls say to me, "I can't get below a certain weight, no matter how hard I try." Of course you can get below a certain weight, but it is a matter of putting in a lot of time and effort. The more you yo-yo, the harder it is for you to achieve any weight loss, much less rapid weight loss.

Why Does Dieting Give Me Bad Breath?

Bad breath in dieting has little to do with the cleanliness of your mouth. You can brush and brush, and the odor doesn't go away. There are several reasons for this problem. When you cut down on your eating, you don't create as much saliva in your mouth. Bacteria tends to stay between the teeth and under the gums. A water pick in addition to brushing your teeth is helpful in getting rid of some of it.

The second cause of bad breath is the hydrochloric acid (HCl) in your stomach. As your stomach contracts, it signals hunger and then releases HCl for digestion. This is the first time you have allowed your stomach to contract and have not fed it. This undiluted hydrochloric acid can often cause unpleasant mouth odors.

The third and most common reason for bad breath is ketosis. When you diet, you have high levels of unburned fatty acids (ketones) in the bloodstream. As the blood circulates into the lungs, the heavy, acid odor of ketones permeates the breath.

The solution for the second and third reasons for bad breath is to take a pleasant-flavored antacid—Mylanta, Gelusil, Tums. These will neutralize your stomach acids and keep the saliva flowing.

Why Do I Get So Many Bruises When I'm Dieting?

Your liver plays a key role in breaking down estrogen. When you diet, it must also break down large amounts of fat. Sometimes its capacity is too limited to handle both, so it leaves excess estrogen in the blood.

Too much estrogen can weaken the smallest blood vessels (capillaries), which then burst more easily. Since bruising can be caused by broken blood vessels, anything that weakens them will make it easier for you to bruise.

High doses of vitamin C (500 mg daily) will help strengthen the walls of the capillaries.

22

Dieting Is a Family Affair

Mother's Section

As the mother of an overweight daughter, you will be reading this section for one of two reasons: (1) You have bought this book for your daughter because you are concerned about her weight problem, but unsure of how to reach her. Perhaps you have had arguments over the subject of dieting. (2) Your daughter has decided to lose weight, and she has bought the book for herself. She is prepared to make a serious commitment, but needs your understanding and support.

Whatever your reason for reading this section, I want to emphasize the intense and emotionally charged interplay that goes on between a mother and daughter when the daughter diets. I want you to see what you might be doing that could hurt your daughter's chances of being a successful dieter.

Why is the level of feeling so intense between the dieter and her mother? It is because a teen-ager senses your mixed emotions, and she resents them. These emotions and the thoughts they inevitably evoke include:

Anger: She looks like a slob. How can she do this to herself? How can she do this to me? What will my friends think? She has no pride! She's eating to spite me. She knows she's upsetting me.
Guilt: How can I think that? She can't help it. It's not her fault. There's something wrong with her glands.

Intense Desire: God! How I wish she was thin like Lynn's kids. She'd be so happy. The phone would be ringing. I'd give anything in the world if she'd lose weight. She's just got to!
Guilt: I'm so selfish. I should be grateful she's not sick or crippled. What am I so upset about? She's a healthy child. Thank God!

Pity: Poor kid. What a bum deal. She's built just like Bernie's mother. She'll never be thin. I wonder who'll marry her. How could anyone fall in love with her?
Guilt: She's a great girl. Anyone with any sense would adore her. She's too good for any of those boys at her school anyway. She needs somebody more mature to appreciate her.

Self Pity: I really needed this—to have a fat kid. Where am I ever going to find a graduation dress to fit her?
Guilt: How can you talk like that? I'll find something and she'll look beautiful. She has such pretty hair, skin, eyes ...

Firmness: No fattening food in this house. No sweets. No chocolate. Just good food. I'm sick of her eating all this junk. We're running a tight ship from now on.
Guilt: Gee, I've got to make her favorite baked stuffed potato for her birthday, and how can I not have a cake? How can I deprive her of all the things she likes. Just a taste won't hurt!

How do most mothers cope with this bewildering mixture of emotions? They cope by "*undoing.*" This is a process by which you try to undo all your bad thoughts with good actions. An example of "physical undoing" is when you buy your daughter the prettiest things you can find and get her the most stylish haircut in town. This is pure self-indulgence.

"Mental undoing" is even more dangerous and insidious. This includes (1) The Blame Game and (2) Overprotection.

(1) *The Blame Game* relies on rationalization or excuse making:

"She's not to blame for her weight because she had no chance. She was a 'preemie' (premature baby) and I fed her too much."

"It was her father's fault because we argued all the time when she was growing up."

"It's the pediatrician's fault; he should have told us she was getting fat."

"It's the school's fault because they have those fattening meals."

"It's all those skinny friends of hers who always try to feed her."

The following is an actual conversation that took place in my office:

Me (to daughter): Why didn't you lose weight this week?
Mother: We went to visit relatives, and it was *impossible* for her to diet.
Me (to daughter); Well, why can't you diet at a relative's house?
Daughter: I ...
Mother: You can't do things like that with family.
Me (to daughter): But must you eat everything that's served to you?
Mother: She didn't want to insult her relatives, and besides ... it was a holiday.

Not a week goes by when I do not see some sort of *undoing* going on in my office. Mothers' excuses for their daughters' breaking a diet often are unbelievably elaborate. She had to eat because ...

"Her grandmother has a bad heart, and we didn't want to aggravate her."

"We went to a restaurant and paid for so much food—and I was darned if she wasn't going to eat it."

"She was studying very hard and needed the energy."

Undoing takes responsibility away from the teen-ager and interferes with her ability to make decisions about when and what she should eat. It can hinder your daughter's emotional growth. In addition, she will use these same excuses her whole life and will never deal honestly with her weight.

(2) *Overprotection.* Many fat girls are emotionally two to three years younger than their chronological ages. They are nice kids, make good baby sitters (and this often is their whole social life), and are quite content to stay as close as possible to the family. To venture out means facing possible disapproval or even scorn. So little girls remain little girls and mothers protect them. They are not exposed to the kinds of crisis situations that are necessary for real growth. Dieting is just another step in personal growth; it requires dedication, commitment, honesty, and perseverance in the face of problems. It requires that a girl constantly reject immediate goals for long-term goals. Dieting is a learning experience.

It is not possible to eliminate your feelings completely, but it *is* possible to understand them and not overreact. If you can become aware of each time you act in an inappropriate way, you will gradually realize how destructive it can be.

Should I Tell My Daughter That She's Fat?

A few days ago a pretty but overweight teen-age girl sat in my office sulking over a 25-pound weight gain. "I want to lose weight, and I want to lose it fast," she pouted. "I want to go back to being normal."

Normal. The word jarred me. To her, normal meant slinking around in beautiful clothes and string bikinis; but, also going out with friends for ice cream sodas and pizza, munching on potato chips and pretzels at parties, and indulging herself in sumptuous dinners and scrumptious desserts.

I decided to be forthright. "You are a fat girl," I said. "And you have the potential to get fatter. There will be no miracle diets and no permanent cures. You'll need a diet to lose weight and a diet to maintain your weight. If you want to be thin, you'll have to change your present eating habits and watch what you eat for the rest of your life."

I was unprepared for her reaction to my "sermon." It began with a single tear rolling down her nose and swelled to a series of heartbreaking sobs. I felt like a heel.

That night, I received a panic-stricken phone call from her mother. "What did you do to my daughter?" she demanded. "She's been crying ever since she got home from your office. She is so depressed that she won't even speak to me."

I felt annoyed at this mother. I was doing *her* job, a job that she was too upset, too uncomfortable, or too ignorant to do: telling her daughter the truth.

Most mothers have difficulty coping with their feelings while watching adolescent daughters eat too much. Their dilemma is how to help an unhappy girl with a weight problem who resents them for trying to help. Most of the time they solve this dilemma by doing nothing and allowing the problem to get—quite frankly—bigger and bigger. No one wants to tell these girls the truth; everyone want them to believe that this bothersome problem will go away with time, once they get "old and smart."

It gets worse with time. "She might grow taller," you think, optimistically. But if she has had her first period, pediatricians tell us that she will not grow much more than an additional two inches. It is estimated that for every one inch of height, a girl can add four to five pounds of weight, depending on her build. Therefore, if she is ten pounds overweight and still has not had her period, she has a chance of "growing out" of her fat. But her weight will continue to climb upward.

Every week in my office, I see former teen-age patients—now in their early twenties. I warned them when I first saw them that their weight would creep up again if they didn't accept the fact that they had a lifetime problem. They assured me that they would *never* get fat again. Yet four to five years later, here they are 15 to 20 to 25 pounds heavier.

"If I bring up my daughter's weight, I'll hurt her feelings," many parents whine. That is like the parents who refuse to discuss suicide with a depressed youngster because they don't want to put the idea of suicide into the child's mind. The kids have the idea anyway, but the parents just don't want to admit it. Overweight girls know that they are overweight. In some cases they might be immature, but they're not stupid, and the refusal on the part of the parent to discuss it only feeds into the teen-ager's own future denials and rationalizations.

Pretend for a moment that your child has a chronic disease that requires certain precautions—precautions that are difficult and often unpleasant and that make her different from the rest of the kids. Take, for instance, the child with little or no protective pigment in her skin who must avoid exposure to direct sunlight. The consequence of going into the sun is not only severe sunburn, but the possibility of skin infections in later life. Would you explain her problem to her or pretend that it doesn't exist? You wouldn't hesitate to tell her! She might cry a few nights or gripe or sulk. She could even say, "To hell with it," and get burned a few times. But sooner or later she would realize that it is foolish to deny something she can't change. She would survive. She would incorporate the difference into her personality, and she would grow. This is the attitude you must take when you're telling a child that for the rest of her life she is going to have to be careful of what she eats if she wants to be thin.

Once you've determined that your child is overweight by objective criteria, which are the scale (most overweight teens won't admit their weight or won't even look at the scale) or weight charts, it is a good idea to have a heart-to-heart talk. When I grew up, it was always a big deal to tell the kids the facts of life. Well, who said the facts of life should be limited to sex? Overweight is certainly a fact of life. You *must* confront your youngster with the fact that she is heavy.

Sit down and talk *with* her—not at her. Give yourself plenty of time, away from the other kids, away from the telephone. Get some information from her. Most overweight teen-agers will not talk freely about the subject. When I visited several area schools, I noticed that thin teen-agers were totally preoccupied with their weight; but the heavier the girls were, the less they were willing to discuss it.

Tell her that you think she has a weight problem. Ask her how she feels about it. Has it ever interfered with anything that she wanted to do? Make it clear to her that if she doesn't want to talk about it, you won't say anything again until she brings it up. But try to persuade her to open up to you.

Don't be surprised if she tells you that she is perfectly happy, that she doesn't mind her weight, that she can do anything she wants to do with the body she has. She might point out that she has plenty of friends, is doing well in school, and that the whole conversation is making her uncomfortable. She might say, "I like to eat, so bug off!"

In this case, you have no recourse but to honor your promise and keep quiet. The timing of the conversation might be off. Perhaps it is too early and she is not ready to accept the responsibility of dieting. But she will remember what she said and—one hopes—the lines of communication will be open. When she does decide to do something about her weight, she will feel that she can come to you for help.

After you have taken the big step, what role should you play in your daughter's diet? You can make things a lot easier by your attitude and support during this difficult time. You should be passive, sympathetic, knowledgeable, and anticipatory.

Passive—no phrases like "Is that on your diet?" or any equally incendiary remarks.

Sympathetic—understand how difficult it is to pass up food that you like.

Knowledgeable—know food, nutrition, and diet. Don't argue that soybeans are healthy when they contain 500 calories a cup. Healthy, yes, but diet food, no.

Anticipatory—it is extremely important for mothers to anticipate problem times for daughters—a bad day at school, a prom she wasn't asked to, and so on. Also, be aware of periods where hunger levels are the highest (after school, for example), and be prepared with low-calorie food.

Food

Much of what you do in the home revolves around the preparation and serving of *food*. Concern yourself with:

1. Appearance of food
2. Quantity
3. Order of serving and time spent eating
4. Availability
5. Nutrition

1. *Appearance of food.* Pay more attention to how food looks. There is something unsavory about a plate that is all light tan or light yellow. Don't be afraid to add a little low-calorie color—watercress, pimento, parsley, scallions, a slice of orange or cherry tomatoes (forget about maraschino cherries, though—they are are much too high in calories).

An aunt of mine used to make food attractive for her little son who was a finicky eater. She made creamy scrambled eggs and shaped them into a circle. She then scooped out holes for eyes, nose, and mouth and filled each hole with creamed spinach. Did you go through all that trouble to make your daughter eat when she was a small child? If it's not too much trouble to fuss over a baby's diet, it shouldn't be too much trouble to fuss over a teen-ager's diet. (Needless to say, don't make funny faces with the scrambled eggs or she'll think you're making fun of her.)

2. *Quantity.* "How can I satisfy an enormous appetite without using starch or filler?" mothers ask. Interestingly enough, as carbohydrate supplies are cut down, enormous appetites diminish, too. Food should be served in individual portions, not family style. Weigh portions to learn how heavy a chicken breast or beef fillet is. You could be giving your daughter a 10-ounce, 1,000-calorie steak and wondering why she isn't losing weight.

Don't cook too much food. A patient of mine recently complained that it was difficult for her to diet because her mother cooked enough food for an army. Therefore, everyone was expected to take second helpings.

3. *Order of serving and time spent eating.* You should also take advantage of the fact that there is a 20-minute lag between the stomach registering "full" and the brain getting the message. Slow down mealtime:

Serve an appetizer. It takes the edge off the appetite. It might be half a grapefruit, a cup of clear soup, salad, or a glass of tomato or low-calorie cranberry juice.

Make meals relaxing. Dinner should be leisurely and geared to conversation with the dieter, even if the rest of the family eats on the run. It's a good idea not to let her eat alone because she often gulps food down without realizing what she is eating.

4. *Availability.* One of the most common reasons for breaking a diet is the absence of low-calorie foods in a home. Sometimes girls tell me, "My family can't afford to keep me on a diet." That is being penny-wise and pound-foolish (pun intended).

You will spend hundreds of dollars getting your child thin during the next eight to ten years. To worry about the cost of food on a normal weight loss diet is senseless. Too many mothers are frightened by crash diets designed for rich suburban housewives, where money is no object and steak or lamb chops are the main protein source. One can diet on hamburger and eggs.

Another complaint I frequently hear is "Somebody ate my diet food." Diet food should not be so special that it becomes the object of everybody's desire. It should be plain, simple, nutritious food, available in adequate supply for whoever wants it. If the family wants diet salad dressing, then use diet dressing for everybody—so no one can "take it" from the dieter.

Learn to substitute if you must. Here are some practical solutions if you run out of diet drinks: suggest club soda or Perrier water with lime, iced decaffeinated coffee with nonfat milk, nonfat milk by itself, homemade lemonade with artificial sweetener, tomato or any other low-calorie juice (not orange). If all else fails, drink just water.

One should not drink excessive amounts of fruit juice because it is high in carbohydrates. But if the choice is between that or regular soda, naturally it's best to have fruit juice (diluted with lots of ice, please). Fresh fruit is also a good thirst quencher, particularly grapefruit.

5. *Nutritional knowledge.* In one school I visited, a little girl told me that her mother was very careful about her diet and always gave her kidney beans instead of potatoes. What that mother didn't realize is that kidney beans have almost three times the calories of potatoes. Remember, there is a difference between what is nutritious and what will make you lose weight. Some suggestions:

Don't serve peas and potatoes together—both are high-starch vegetables. If you can't be more imaginative, leave one out.

Don't serve 200 calories worth of butter on 100 calories worth of vegetables.

Don't think that only expensive meat is good for dieting. Actually, the toughest, cheapest cuts of beef are far better for a diet than a tender steak riddled with fat. You never have to see a piece of lamb to go on an effective diet.

The least expensive animal protein is the best for dieting: chicken. Ounce for ounce you get more protein and less fat for your money. Eggs and cottage cheese are also low-cost, high-protein foods, and if the budget doesn't allow for meat, they are far better to use than moderate-protein, high-starch beans.

Many mothers complain about the cost of lettuce for salads. If you don't want to pay ninety-nine cents for a head of lettuce, buy five cucumbers for a dollar. With a little imagination, you can make marvelous, low-cost salads anytime. Just watch for sales and buy the cheapest produce. You will be amazed at the number of vegetables with which you can create a salad. When all else fails, you can resort to the two-bean salad made with yellow and green beans, onion, celery, vinegar, and low-calorie sweetener.

If you must use starch as a filler, keep it plain: baked potato with salt (100 calories) or a cup of plain white rice (161 calories). Don't make fillers too interesting. You'll add more calories and encourage the dieter to eat more.

Don't say things like, "Fruit is fattening." It might slow down weight loss, but it beats the sugary alternative.

Don't worry about too much low-calorie liquid ("She drinks gallons of water") or too much salt ("She ate a whole jar of dill pickles yesterday"). If these things do give rise to fluid retention, it is not that significant in the teen-ager. Besides, they take up volume—and that is an important consideration in dieting.

This list is just a tiny sample of the kinds of common nutritional mistakes that mothers make. Also, it illustrates some of the faulty thinking that still goes on about dieting.

By now I have probably lost some irate mothers, who grumble, "Why me? Why do I have to do all this work? I mean, she's almost an adult." The "almost" is a very big word. You have kept her a baby, warned her of all the dangers in this world, criticized her first date (if she had one), scrutinized her friends, passed judgment on her teachers, monitored her phone calls, enforced her bedtime, shopped with her for clothes, and now you call her an adult when it comes to feeding herself. Curious!

This is the beginning of a particular growing process; let's call it nutritional growth. Are you helping her to grow nutritionally? Or do you shove her into the kitchen just to do the dishes or set the table and ignore her suggestions about meal planning? Do you give her a list of foods to buy at the supermarket, with stern instructions not to buy one more thing? If you've done these things, don't suddenly decide that she is grown up where food is concerned.

Once you take the position of helping a dieter, you should follow through. If you are going to encourage your daughter to diet, don't be inconsistent. *Don't* say, "Take this, it won't hurt you." Most dieters cannot be too fanatical about sticking to their diet (except for anorexics). That's what makes them successful. Don't get angry because your child refuses something that is not on her diet. Be proud of her determination.

Don't be a mother who says, "But I have the rest of the family to feed. I can't be concerned with just her." I always ask that mother what she would do if somebody in the family were an alcoholic: put a bottle on the table and invite the rest of the family to have a drink? Most mothers are horrified at the suggestion.

It is extremely important not to put food on the table that is particularly tempting to the dieting teen-ager. *Reducing* diets do have a beginning and an end; the family can bear the "hardship" for a short time. The others will just have to eat their goodies outside the house. Thin people have the option of getting high-calorie foods anywhere, anyplace, anytime. Besides, nobody *needs* the kind of high-carbohydrate foods that make people fat.

Don't think food is equal to love. Every time you bake a birthday cake or cook special food for the child who is home from college you are saying, "I do this because I love you and I want to see you happy." A mother of an overweight daughter would be better off showing her love in other ways.

Don't be uptight about meals. What if your child eats only hamburger, string beans, skim milk, and oranges? Serve her hamburger, string beans, skim milk, and oranges. They are good diet foods, nutritious, and well-balanced. You might want to get variety into her diet, but if you can't, don't worry—eating the same foods is only a problem if your daughter claims to be bored.

When she shows signs of boredom, suggest different foods for her to try. Watch out for the word "bored" though; even in the most compliant dieters, it could be the first sign of trouble. Dieters frequently use boredom as an excuse to eat larger amounts of carbohydrates.

Don't feed a cold. "What happens when she's sick?" many of my patients' mothers ask me. "Shouldn't she have more food?" No! When you have too much body fat, that fat supplies you with emergency fuel. Food has no curative value. (Although recent studies conclude that chicken soup unclogs noses.) Be realistic about the kind of food she needs, depending on her ailment. Chances are it doesn't have to be high in calories.

If you start "feeding a cold" in a dieting teen-ager, you will just awaken her desire to overeat. *Remember, almost any dieter will eat if you push her hard enough.*

The best advice I can give to mothers of dieting daughters is to treat them as most wives treat their husbands who diet for their health: compliance, silence, and approval. I rarely see a wife sabotage her husband's diet. When husbands diet, the whole family diets; when a child diets, she diets alone.

Exercise

Before you try to start your daughter on an exercise program, give her an exercise assessment test. First, check to make sure that she has no physical problem that will get in the way of her exercising. I have seen girls with curvature of the spine whose mothers pushed them to do exercises that were not good for them. It wasn't until the girls experienced pain that this defect was found. It is a good idea to have your doctor's okay for all physical activities.

Consider stamina and build when planning an exercise program. Muscular girls do much better in sports that require sustained energy release, like rowing, swimming, long-distance running. Slender girls do better in calisthenics, figure skating, and dancing. Overweight girls in general do better in spurt sports (ones where you can start and stop, like volleyball, basketball, and softball). There are exceptions to all these rules, however.

Make sure that when a child enters into a sport, she has some feeling for it. It is damaging to force somebody into a situation that they can't cope with, let alone master. I have seen fathers try to make football stars out of their sons when these boys were totally incapable of playing the game and have seen mothers force daughters to dance when the girls lacked grace and agility and even disliked it.

Call the physical education instructor at your daughter's school and ask if there are any areas in which she is particularly interested or shows some ability. Some girls won't seem physically fit for anything. They should be eased into any exercise situation.

There are the girls we call accident-prone (the klutz or the kid who trips over her own feet). Psychiatrists tell us that these people do not really want to do what they are doing; their accidents are a form of resistance acted-out rather than verbalized.

Exercise should not end with the school year—the patterns established should be lifelong. It doesn't matter if the only sport in which your daughter excels is Ping-Pong. Pursue it! Subscribe to a Ping-Pong magazine, have her join a Ping-Pong club, go to Ping-Pong tournaments—if that is what she likes.

Consider income level when encouraging a child to attempt a sport. If you can't afford it and there's no cheap way to do it, forget it. Some sports are costly. Downhill skiing, for example, has priced itself out of the average teen-ager's pocketbook. Cross-country skiing is taking its place. You get more exercise, it's cheaper, and the family can do it together. Another plus is that you don't have to travel very far to participate—any flat piece of land can be converted into a site for cross-country skiing.

Golf is an expensive sport, unless your town has a public golf course and offers free instruction.

Tennis can be reasonable if you live in an area where there are a number of public tennis courts. Park systems sometimes offer free tennis lessons.

Investigate community resources, if income is a problem, to find out what facilities your town offers. Some towns promote Little League teams. These used to be all male, but lately girls are competing for team spots. Our community center offers a "Biddy Basketball" for kids not old enough to be on regular basketball teams. Girls are now included in that sport.

Presently, sports scholarships are not widely available to women, but this is changing. Naturally, the best-paying scholarships are awarded to male football and basketball players, but in the future, excellence in sports may open up many educational doors for women.

One of my friend's daughters, who is very proficient in lacrosse, has been approached by several colleges. Sports such as rowing, tennis, golf, and even basketball have been assuming more importance to females, and there is now more scholarship money being put aside for them.

Skills and Hobbies

Skills and hobbies can be educational and fun, and they also can take a bored teen-ager's mind off eating. If your daughter has too much free time in which to eat, suggest she cultivate a skill or find a hobby.

Most girls have some kind of talent. Sometimes you have to uncover it. You might hear your daughter singing and suddenly realize that she has a very nice voice. You might discover that she has perfect pitch and would love to play an instrument. However, as in athletics, you must be extremely careful not to push a teen-ager into something she doesn't want to do, or even worse, to overestimate her talent.

Hobbies are quite different. They provide enjoyment and relaxation. Common hobbies include collecting everything from stamps to comic books, knitting, needlepoint, sewing, model-building, and more. Sometimes hobbies can become financially rewarding.

Seeking Help Outside the Home

Sometimes, you can only do so much by yourself—either because you are too emotionally involved or too confused to know what is right. You might also be worried that you are doing the wrong thing and need reassurance. This is when it's time to take Operation Diet outside of the house.

The most logical first step is to take your daughter to her pediatrician. This could get you nowhere. With a slap on the fanny or friendly hug, the doctor could say, "Don't worry about her. When she starts to like boys, she will get thin." If she waits until she notices boys to start to slim down, boys might not notice her. This could make her so unhappy that she would eat more out of frustration.

Or perhaps he will shrug and say, "This is baby fat and she will outgrow it." LITTLE GIRLS RARELY OUTGROW BABY FAT! The baby fat that they have at adolescence is there to stay unless they do something about it. Your son can outgrow his baby fat, but daughters must take definite steps to diet or they will have a weight problem for a long, long time.

Suppose your doctor listens to you, is sympathetic, and tries to help. What can he do? He can't diet for your daughter. Don't expect him to provide miracles. This is a special type of medicine. Since I wrote my last book, I have been seeing many patients from distant cities. Naturally, this is flattering, but it is not logical. As capable, knowledgeable, and caring as I might be, I work no medical magic. My patient is the most important ingredient in my success. In other words, a successful outcome of a diet depends upon a cooperative, well-motivated patient. A good doctor can be exceedingly helpful, but he or she alone is not the answer.

What exactly can doctors be expected to do for a dieting youngster?

1. *They can rule out the presence of physical disease.* Only a small number of overweights prove to have a glandular or thyroid problem, but most mothers like to have their daughters' thyroid checked anyway. I know doctors who refuse to order thyroid blood tests because they claim to *know* that nothing is wrong. Nobody should be deprived of the right to have a blood test, if for no other reason than to keep the parents from becoming anxious.

2. *They can interpret laboratory blood tests.* They don't scare people if minor abnormalities exist. They are able to correlate the lab studies with what is clinically going on in the patient. For example, low blood sugar does not necessarily mean that the patient has hypoglycemia, if there are no other symptoms present.

3. *They can evaluate the degree of overweight and evaluate medical or psychiatric problems that might hinder effective dieting.* If they find either, they try to correct it before initiating any diet.

4. *They assess diet readiness.* Perhaps the child is too immature to understand the responsibility of this kind of commitment and will only fail and frustrate herself. At this point, doctors take a "holding" position. They wait until they can work through the problem with the patient, explaining that there might be a better time for her to diet. They must do this in such a way as not to discourage her from future

attempts. They must also try, if possible, to prevent her from gaining any more weight.

5. *They can devise a realistic exercise program.* In the course of a physical exam, doctors recognize physical defects that could lead to problems, even in a mild exercise program. For example, there could be an anatomic abnormality of the knee that would make it difficult for the teen-ager to do certain kinds of exercise. She might be the kind of person who could never do gymnastics, but could participate in regular calisthenics that don't require stretching or twisting.

6. *They can weed out any suspected allergies or peculiarities that are related to food.* Some of the allergies (see Allergies, Chapter 15) often give rise to bizarre symptoms that are frequently mistaken for more serious physical ailments.

7. *They are able to interpret physical changes and problems that occur during and after a diet.* When these problems occur, they will determine which are routine and which are serious, which are diet-connected and which are not. Periods might go haywire, becoming excessive or scanty. There may be hair loss, dry skin, and strange rashes. Are they dangerous or just annoying? Should you worry or relax? Physicians help you through these trying periods.

I feel that medical doctors are in an extremely unique position to oversee dieting, if they want to. There is no question that overweight is a metabolic disease. Whether or not it is related to thyroid is unclear. Obviously, the difference between thin and fat people goes beyond the mere intake of food and output of activity.

When I went to medical school, there was no nutritional training for physicians. However, I recently attended four major postgraduate conferences that dealt with the subject of nutrition, diet, and obesity. Medical schools have been a little slow in organizing a curriculum in nutrition, but these postgraduate courses have been excellent. Medical nutrition is now a recognized and growing field that concentrates not only on overnutrition (obesity), but on nutrition in relation to disease, healing, and longevity. Therefore, the most logical first step that a mother can take for her child is to have her evaluated by a physician.

Whatever decision she makes after that will at least be *informed.* Once you have done all you can by yourself, enlisted the aid of your pediatrician, and encouraged your daughter to read this book, there are still alternatives to be considered.

Diet Camps

As much as I am against incarceration for dieting, either anatomic (like mouth wiring) or geographic (like going to Duke University to be put on the famous rice diet), I think that a diet camp may have an important place in the treatment of the overweight adolescent.

A well-run diet camp can be the ideal place in which to initiate a diet and to develop—out of necessity—better eating habits. Exercising is also strongly encouraged, but here the competition isn't so trim and experienced. There are gab sessions where a girl can interact with others of her own age with many of her own problems. Finally, a diet camp is the one place that will cater to all her dieting needs (for a price, of course, and, unfortunately, it costs a lot of money).

The problem is that the girl must return to the real world, where cooperation is not as ideal and temptations are many. But as long as the camp prepares the camper for this transition, it is doing its job. If a youngster returns to civilization thinking that the whole world is like a diet camp, she is in for a big disappointment.

Why do I, a progressive physician, think that diet camps—so often portrayed as medieval prisons—are good places for teen-agers? No, I don't run one. The answer has to do with age. When we physicians treat adults, we are trying to reprogram them to break a lifetime of wrong attitudes and fixed behaviors. The results have generally been poor. With teen-agers, the focus is on education for *prevention*. Furthermore, after some initial adjustment problems, many overweight girls have wonderful times at summer camp.

Check the credentials on any diet camp with the American Camping Association and make sure that it is well-run and financially solvent. I have read horror stories about camps closing in midsummer and stranding the campers. (My son almost went to one of them.) More important, have your daughter talk to several people who have been to the camp. They can tell you if the staff is considerate and aware and if the exercise program is consistent and practical. Brochures, unfortunately, don't tell everything.

Psychiatrists

Psychiatrists have been very cautious in treating overweight teen-agers. They only want to uncover the emotional problems that led to the weight gain and often neglect the practical problem of excessive adipose tissue. The psychiatrist rationalizes by saying, "If I take care of what's bothering her, the weight will take care of itself." That doesn't happen. You have to take care of both problems.

A psychiatrist isn't a bad idea for your daughter if she is interested in understanding some of her defenses. There is nothing wrong with allowing a teen-age girl a few sessions to talk with somebody who can look at her problems objectively (and everybody at this age has some problems). It's about time that we rid ourselves of the notion that psychiatrists are only for crazy people.

Unfortunately, the price tag is high. Taken in the proper perspective, however, it is no higher than diet camps or any other diet advice that you will purchase for the rest of your teen-ager's overweight existence. Curing overweight can be very expensive.

My gripe with psychiatrists is that they take too long to do too little. Pathological or sick overeating is *not* the most common reason for a teen-ager to gain weight. Genetic and environmental reasons are just as important as emotional ones. All of these things, *plus* the availability of high-calorie, tempting food, lead to obesity. Taking care of one without understanding the other will be of little value in the overall treatment of overweight.

In addition to individual psychiatric treatment, many local groups are currently forming around the country for overweight adolescents to discuss their feelings about being overweight. These groups give excellent emotional support, but often are poorly focused in the practical nutritional area.

Father's Section

Fathers rarely exert a positive influence on their daughters' weight-loss programs. They could play an active part, but they often don't want to hurt their daughters' feelings. Besides, they want their daughters to love them, and it's very difficult to set limits when you're worried about losing love. But a weight problem can cause a lot of future pain and unhappiness; if you could see that, you would probably want to help your daughter *now*. Here are some things that you can do to assist her diet:

1. Don't insist on lots of starches and high-calorie foods at meals. Eat big lunches and accept low-calorie suppers graciously.

2. Try not to bring home pastries and candies. If you want those things, keep them in the car. If you must bring them inside, hide them in your bedroom.

3. If you are taking the family out to dinner, give the kid a break. Avoid places that serve only fried foods. If there is a money problem, there are plenty of cheap steak houses that have salad bars. If you must go to a place where your daughter cannot buy appropriate food—a pizza parlor, for example—do her a favor and let her stay home.

4. Ask you wife not to stock up on junk food in the house. With your approval she is apt to take things more seriously.

5. Every so often buy your daughter something pretty to wear—to show that you notice what she is doing and appreciate her hard work. I know many fathers who promise their daughters whole wardrobes if they succeed in losing weight. (You don't have to be *that* lavish, but you get the idea.)

6. Develop a better relationship. Offer to take walks with her at night and/or jog with her in the morning. She does enough with her mother; now it's your turn. Since she may be less resentful of you, try to get her to talk about her weight and about any problems she might be having. Inquire if there is anything you can do at home to make it easier for her. Get involved in her efforts to develop new skills, hobbies, or interests that will keep her mind off food. If your daughter enjoys one of your favorite sports—skiing or skating, for example—be sure to make plans to take her away for the day. Bring her to work if you can. Make her feel that she is an important part of your life.

7. If you are divorced and have only visiting privileges, make the time you spend together as active as possible or make it a "low-calorie weekend." She could even lose a few pounds in the time she spends with you. If you remarry, you should discuss the problem with your new wife so that she can plan her menu accordingly when your daughter comes to visit.

This section is shorter than the mother's because mothers still have much more control over their daughters. Fathers don't seem to get caught in the tangled psychic web that marks mother-daughter relationships. However, a father-daughter relationship is very special; fathers can exert a positive influence if they want to; sometimes, in fact, a father can do more with a few words than a mother with hours of pleading.

Brothers and Sisters

Brothers can be remarkably insensitive and nasty. Family arguments often break down into name-calling sessions, in which the thin brother needles the heavy sister. "You're a moron," the sister might say, and the brother replies, "You're a fat slob!" This kind of insult, repeated again and again, makes the overweight sister extremely sensitive to the whole subject of fat and food.

Most sisters of dieters are supportive. I heard a very nice story about three sisters who dieted together every spring, after winter had played havoc with their weight. The three planned their menus for a period of six weeks and worked out a complete exercise program.

Brother and/or sisters: Here are some suggestions on how to handle a dieting sister.

1. Don't bring up her excess weight while she's trying to lose it. Nothing makes her more upset than being called a pig if she is eating only 1,000 calories a day. If you have to insult her, insult the size of her feet, her personality, or her IQ, but don't insult her weight.

2. If you know her weakness is chocolate chip cookies and you want some, buy them at the store and keep them in your room during the time she's dieting. Perhaps you like Fig Newtons and she detests them. Then that's the cookie to keep in the house. Don't play into her likes or dislikes.

3. Don't offer her food when she's trying to resist temptation. Don't leave candy, cake, or any other kind of munchies lying around. After you finish eating something, close the package carefully and put it away in a spot where she will not be likely to see it the minute she comes into the house.

4. Don't remind her that she's on a diet if she snitches a piece of candy or a cookie. This will only upset her and probably cause her to eat more. She is going to have to take an adult's responsibility for what she puts into her own mouth.

5. Compliment her as she loses weight. That doesn't mean you should pretend to recognize small differences in size. Don't be too nice—she'll know it's phony. But if you *do* notice something, don't keep silent.

6. Be a friend and get her mind off food. Include her in plans if she has nothing else to do. Sitting around the house alone is an excellent way to start nibbling. Chances are she won't go with you, but she'll appreciate the invitation.

7. Don't give her candy or food if the occasion demands a present. Give her a tube of lipstick, a pretty scarf, or some of that cute, inexpensive fashion jewelry that won't put a dent in your budget.

8. And most important, if she doesn't succeed, don't make life miserable for her. Accept her as she is and appreciate her other good qualities. In dieting, "Today is the first day of the rest of your life," and who knows, the next time she starts to diet, she might be more successful.

Grandmothers and Grandfathers

I once overheard a grandmother say, "I don't understand the way my daughter-in-law feeds that child. She watches everything the poor kid puts in her mouth. I think it's terrible." You know what's going to happen when that particular child visits her grandmother. The grandmother is going to make sure that the girl has plenty to eat.

Many grandparents set themselves up as the opposites of the parents, so if the parents restrict food intake, the grandparents push food. The implication is, "Look how much I love you because I'm giving you food."

Grandparents are worse than fathers when it comes to evaluating a child realistically. If the father sees his daughter as beautiful in spite of her weight, then grandparents see her as *just* beautiful.

Grandparents must realize that the overweight child can lead an unhappy and sometimes miserable life because she weighs too much. It is not in the child's best interest for grandparents to offer her foods that will make losing weight more difficult.

Here are some rules that grandparents should follow if they have a grandchild with a weight problem.

1. Don't cook fattening foods for them. Keep it simple and keep it plain.

2. Don't feel hurt if your granddaughter refuses to eat something you cooked because she is on a diet. This is a tragic flaw in grandparents. They make the grandchild feel guilty for not eating. It's tough enough for a dieter to keep on a diet without having a loved one raise all kinds of psychological conflicts.

3. Don't take sides with the grandchild against her mother. It will create a lot of hard feelings and obscure the most important issue, which is keeping the teen-ager on a diet.

4. Do ask a visiting grandchild what *she* would like to eat while she's visiting.

5. Do ask a visiting grandchild to help with the shopping and the meal preparation.

6. Don't tell your grandchild that she is *too* thin if she looks thinner to you. Don't tell your grandchild that she will get sick if she doesn't eat.

7. Try to understand that you are doing her a favor if you help her stay on a diet.

Remember, normal children usually do not harm their bodies by dieting. Crash dieting is usually short-lived because the dieter gets tired of it. Sensible dieting is the most healthy thing that anybody with a weight problem can do.

The Family Meeting

Every dieter should have the right to call a family meeting. The purpose of the meeting is for her to discuss with members of the family what she is trying to accomplish. It should be a free exchange of ideas. It might put some stress on the dieter, but a family meeting lacking in honesty has no value.

A mother should feel free to say that she doesn't know how she can find the time and/or the money to prepare special foods for her daughter's diet. A father can feel free to say that he has no particular interest in what's going on and, therefore, he's not going to contribute much. Brothers and sisters might say they think the whole idea is silly and a waste of time.

In the initial family meeting, the dieter might say, "I intend to give up all refined sugar. I'm interested in seeing how effective this will be. I'll eat fresh or frozen food only. I hope nobody objects." At this point mother might say, "I think that's a ridiculous way for you to diet because you're not going to lose any weight." Or, "We don't have enough space in the freezer to stock up on frozen vegetables." Or, "I don't feel like preparing fresh vegetables." The teen-ager could become angry with her mother for not wanting to take the time for special preparation, or she can volunteer to do the extra work to provide for her diet herself.

A teen-ager might also tell the family, "I am only going to diet for two weeks and I want to go on a crash diet. I'm only going to drink fruit juices and take vitamin pills." Her father might say, "You're not going to do anything of the sort. I think that's a very unhealthy way to diet and I will not go along with it."

The family might point out that there is a schedule problem that makes a diet impractical at this time. Perhaps they are taking the family to the beach for the summer, where there is limited food storage space and no one wants to cook. The dieter could suggest a compromise. She could say she's willing to shop for small amounts of food every day and to do her own cooking.

The first step at the family meeting is to assess the reality of any given diet. Discuss how practical it will be to follow.

Arrange for future meetings. Between meetings, all members of the family should hold their comments and write them down, to be aired at the next meeting. Comments might include resentment created because siblings feel that the dieter is getting too much attention. Talk about it! Some member of the family might point out that the dieter seemed to be using excessive amounts of salad dressing or eating too much fruit. Bring it up. The dieter should not become angry or resentful. Take the suggestions, evaluate them, and respond. This is not an excuse for a family argument. It is an exchange of ideas and feelings.

At the conclusion of a diet, whether it's natural (because she's lost all her excess weight) or the bitter end (because she prefers not to diet anymore), she has a right to call a moratorium on the family sessions. At that time an emergency session can be called and she can state, "I am no longer dieting because..." and then can give the reason: "I don't feel like it" or "It's making me sick." On the other hand, if the diet is progressing well, it might be nice for the dieter to give a progress report, which includes number of pounds lost, whether or not she is satisfied, and her feelings about the diet at this particular stage.

The most successful family meetings involve the *core* family, the mother, father, and brothers and/or sisters. However, if there are any real problems, the dieter can invite close relatives, particularly grandparents or aunts and uncles. Many dieters like to invite friends to the meeting, particularly friends in whom they confide.

There should be a firm rule that no information leave the family meeting. What is discussed at that meeting is what doctors call "privileged communication." That means it's there for the ears of the participants and should go no further. This information should never be brought up in anger or in spite. These are private feelings voiced in an effort to bring the dieter and her family together to work toward the same goal.

23

The Right to Be Overweight

A recent newspaper quoted a well-known expert in adolescent obesity as saying, "Some youngsters will never be thin ... buy clothes that fit them and forget it." Although I devoted two books to the subject of weight loss, I agree with him wholeheartedly. A girl has the right to be overweight.

Some girls will not be able to get thin—for whatever combination of reasons that exist in their lives. There are also girls who do not *want* to get thin, who feel that it's not worth the sacrifice of having to watch every piece of food they put in their mouths. And if that's how they feel, bless them. As long as they are not so obese as to endanger their health, there's no reason for them to suffer because of their appearance.

Many teen-agers tell me, "Fat or thin, you've got to have a feeling of self-worth." Once an overweight girl stops punishing herself and begins to think positively, she becomes far happier and far more successful in life. She might not be delighted about her weight, but she doesn't try to hide because of it. She "accentuates the positive."

It is strange that only *female* body size can create such problems. Recently, at a swanky hotel in Florida, I saw many obese men married to thin women, and no one said a word. I saw one obese woman married to a thin man and everyone said, "How could he have married her?"

In a men's store in the hotel, a very heavy man was being fitted for a pair of pants. The salesperson said nothing. In the same shop, a beautiful young girl was buying a present for her father. The girl was a little chubby, and the same salesperson, who had just silently fitted the overweight man for pants, said to her, "It's a shame you are overweight—you have such a pretty face." If I'd been that girl, I'd have belted him.

You are approaching an age where physical attractiveness is very important. Boys are not judged on appearance—looks can play only a small part in their popularity. They are judged on personality, physical strength, athletic ability, and intelligence. They don't have to be handsome to feel pretty good about themselves. It's rather unfair. If you are overweight or your legs or hips are too big, you have to go around feeling inferior to someone who is *only* thinner than you. Have you ever stopped to think that it's kind of a raw deal?

Who do you think is going to change the kind of thinking that equates feminine worth with physical beauty? Certainly not the fashion designers—they are going to keep pushing, "Thin is beautiful, thin is desirable, thin is the *only* way to be." It is a lot easier to design something fashionable for someone 5 feet 10 inches and 110 pounds than for someone 5 feet 2 inches and 130 pounds. They can also use less material. Fashion designs favor the kind of looks that are going to show off their clothes. They have nothing but contempt for the overweight female. When one designer was asked why he didn't design clothes for overweight females, he responded, "I design dresses, not tents."

People like to think that if you can't succeed in losing weight, you can't succeed in anything else. NONSENSE! If you really wanted to lose weight, you could—but it would take more of an effort than you are currently prepared to make. If the people who criticize your weight had your genetic makeup, chances are they wouldn't think it was so easy to lose weight and such a sign of failure to be fat.

You are going to have to change people's thinking. Make it difficult for society to punish you. Too many overweight girls hide at home, behind their families. It is time you came out of hiding and said, "Look at me! I'm a wonderful person no matter what I weigh. I'll be what I want, I'll dress the way I want, and I will lose weight when I want to." And be good at what you do, so good that people *can't* discriminate against you.

Even if you feel terrible about your weight, don't despair. In dieting, there is always tomorrow. There are no last chances, just new starts. If someday you really want to change your image, you will do it. In the meantime, things could be a lot worse.

Conclusion

I have covered a great deal in this book. The teen-ager growing up in today's world should realize the problems associated with being overweight, as well as the problems associated with weight loss and weight maintenance.

It is imperative to understand that there is no magical way to deal with the problem of obesity. It takes hard work, dedication, and an understanding of nutrition. It takes a sense of pride in one's body that includes a continuing program of exercise and physical fitness. I hope this book will serve as a guide to teen-age girls in any future endeavors that they undertake in relation to dieting.

Index